CyclingWithMS

Ewan Johnston

https://cyclingwithms.wordpress.com/

ISBN: 9781726655026

Foreword

I'm not a writer.

I'm not even a cyclist, not a professional one anyway.

But I do have MS, diagnosed in March 2015.

Since then, I've undergone two bouts of immune-modifying chemotherapy... and have cycled over 45,000 miles.

It's been quite a journey.

To try to organise my own thoughts during this remarkable time, I started to write a diarised blog entitled "CyclingWithMS". I found this exercise enormously therapeutic and was hugely buoyed by the messages of support that it elicited.

As my blog grew and grew, it became harder for readers to find a coherent story so, this year, whilst laid low by ill health, I spent my bedbound time transforming my various diary extracts into a single book.

And here it is.

The result is that the following chapters are not necessarily in chronological order and have had to be heavily edited from their original form but I feel that they now best-represent the trials, tribulations and joys of a life with MS.

I hope that they provide you with an entertaining read.

Contents

Introduction

About me

My name is Ewan Johnston.

I am 41 years old.

For over 20 of those, one thing has been a constant in my life: my love of getting places by bike.

This all started when I was working in London. I would wend my way, firstly, through alleys and backstreets from North London down to Blackfriars, then, latterly, over cobbles and footbridges across to the shining skyscrapers of Canary Wharf.

Since then, I've taken my bike (and it has taken me) to some of my favourite places in the world: I have mountain biked across Iceland and ridden Land's End to John O'Groats; toured the Rhone and the Rhine; and cycled the width of France and the length of the Pyrenees.

When we first met, my (now) wife and I mountain biked around South Wales; cycling became how I met new friends and a part of my identity, representing both what I had done in life and what I wanted to do. Still today, whenever I find myself somewhere new, my first inclination is to explore by bike – only then can I feel comfortable with where I am in the world.

Now based just outside Bristol, married with two young boys, I've recently taken to wheeling us out on family rides around local bike paths and waterways, although it usually falls to me to provide sufficient enthusiasm for all four of us.

I have never been a bike racer but, through various cycling clubs, I've entered (rather slow) time trial events, hill climbs, endurance races and sportives. I've ridden in audaxes, mountain bike marathons, triathlons, charity events and Sunday Club rides... the wheels always turning... always wanting to see around that next corner (always one more...) I used to ride over 5,000 miles a year; then it became six, then seven. In 2013, I cycled over 10 thousand; in 2014, the figure was over 12.

2015 started like any other year. I tried to lift the gloom of winter by making exciting plans for when the days would grow long and the sun would come out again. I had long read about the world-famous Paris-Brest-Paris cycling event that is run in August so I targeted this as the year's ambition. A friend of mine was also keen so, together, a whole series of qualifying events was booked, logistics were organised and aspirations set. I was really excited by the prospect and couldn't wait for summer.

Then, on 18th February 2015, I was hit head-on by a car as I cycled to work. It hurt. Although my bike was obliterated, I had been lucky. Despite being knocked unconscious and needing 44 stitches in various facial wounds, I only broke a single tooth and an index finger. My recovery, however, proved stuttering. I was convinced that I must have damaged my back as I kept getting odd sensory distortions down my legs and unremitting pins and needles in my feet. I was sleeping 14 hours a night and still needing a nap in the day. I was beset by an exhaustion and lethargy that I felt was out of keeping with the injuries I had sustained. Ultimately, my GP advised me to report to A&E.

48 hours later the neurologist registrar at Southmead Hospital was explaining to me that that I was suffering from Multiple Sclerosis.

A game changer.

MS and Jeff Goldblum

Immediately post-diagnosis, I was told to return home and continue with my normal life. As soon as my health issues had a name, all urgency seemed to disappear. My GP would prescribe me medicines to manage my current symptoms and a letter would be in the post with a date for a follow-up appointment with a consultant where all would be explained.

My new normal. My new life.

I googled "MS" and tried not to feel lost at sea.

Day diagnosis-plus-2, I set off on my bike, on my usual downhill ride to work.

I was well aware that I hadn't felt right from the moment I woke up and my body felt badly out of kilter. Of course, it was raining.

Barely a couple of miles from home and I pulled off the road. I had a complete lack of strength in my legs, my arms muscles were buzzing and it felt as though my bike was hardly moving. The rain was cold though, I started shivering almost immediately and my hands were starting to get numb. Through sheer lack of a better idea, I just pointed my bike onwards and carried on.

I felt badly under the weather all day and eventually worked out a way of getting a lift home that evening. I went to bed at 8pm.

Then, the next day, I woke with a start at 4am, buzzing with adrenalin. Eventually, I gave up trying to go back to sleep, crept out of the house and wheeled my bike out of our quiet cul-de-sac before sunrise. I felt strong and rode fast through the clear, bright morning on car-free roads down the hill to work.

Wonderful. And confusing.

When I was a young boy I remember being fascinated with the Guinness World of Records. Of course, the athletic exploits of the likes of Carl Lewis or Bob Beamer were awesome, but it was the human curiosities that led to my real wonderment: the fattest man; the boy who had sneezed continuously for three years; and the woman with the longest fingernails.

The previous fortnight it had seemed like my body was introducing new unnerving symptoms almost daily: I briefly lost partial use of my right hand; three times I lost my sense of balance for a couple of minutes; and the skin on my legs started to go bright pink after a warm shower. I experienced what I think is called "an MS hug": I can only describe this as the feeling that cold water was trickling down my back (I actually thought I'd brushed against something wet). When the sensation spread around my waist, I could only assume that it was just another MS-oddity.

In the classic sci-fi, horror film, "The Fly", Jeff Goldblum (for reasons perhaps best left unexplained) slowly transforms into the insect. The fear that viewers seem to empathise with is his morbid fascination as he slowly witnesses the ghastly metamorphosis that is taking place; a healthy man watching the slow disintegration of his humanity. I poke fun at myself and make this cinematic reference light-heartedly but it was a truly disconcerting couple of weeks for me.

As it turned out, the pins and needles in both legs persisted for three weeks without pause. Beyond that, my left arm continued tingling, as did the weird sensory distortions around my waist. Whenever I tried to ride my bike, I found that I had neither strength nor stamina and my feet hurt as if frozen cold.

Upon diagnosis my GP prescribed, and I consumed, a course of steroids which I seemed to absorb without my body so much as noticing.

I saw my GP, again.

I called a number I'd be given for the MS nurses in Bristol. Frustratingly, the message from them was that the steroids I had been on weren't the best ones, I had been prescribed "Prednisolone" when apparently "Methyprednisolone" might have been better. The strange, emotional, steroidal ups-and-downs I had been experiencing might have been in vain, but when I googled these new drugs, I mixed up their long names and couldn't work out any discernible difference between the two of them anyway.

Levels of sympathy were high but not much could be done. I was told, again, to wait for my follow-up appointment when the MS condition, its symptoms and my prognosis would be better explained.

Chapter One: Diagnosis

Can you cycle with MS? Versus MS?

First off, I very much don't want to die prematurely.

I want to live a long, healthy and full life with zero disability. Thank you.

I have a wife and two sons whom I'm loving watch grow up. I'm self-employed. I love travelling. I love cycling.

We're trying to buy a house.

The sun is shining.

The only thing to do at the moment would seem to be to wait, then let the cogs of the health service, and the condition, turn.

Can you cycle with MS?

I have asked the same question of every healthcare professional that I have seen since diagnosis:

Will cycling in any way worsen my MS condition?

And the answer has always been, "No."

As I get back onto my bike and wobble slightly with weakness, I repeat this to myself.

"No – it will not."

In any given week, I'm usually out on my bike for about 15 hours.

The first advice, offered to me within 10 seconds of my diagnosis, was "of course you can keep cycling, just take it a bit easier."

"I commute to work by bike," I said.

"That should be fine, just go easy if you're feeling tired."
"I'm planning to ride a 200km ride this Saturday," I said.
"Sounds excessive," was the reply.

I search the internet. Advice seems to be MS patients should aim to do three to five half hour sessions of moderate exercise every week (which aligns to advice given to the rest of the population), but that this should vary with capability and fitness. My cyclo-commute is currently one hour each way, Monday to Friday.

I wait for the much-heralded appointment letter to arrive but burn with impatience. I hate the feeling that I sit passively as my MS is left to establish a foothold.

Versus MS?

Another fortnight passes and the next pharmaceutical to be introduced to my system is a pill called "Gabapentine". On balance, this does seem to reduce the throbbing numbness in my legs and feet. The incessant pins and needles that I'd had for almost a month improved from pain to mild discomfort. It felt as though I could walk again without having to adopt hobbling pigeon-steps and suddenly all my other symptoms also seemed much more manageable. Numbness, hypersensitivity and the occasion spasm in my thighs remained but these were completely bearable.

My main concern became the blurry distortion to my vision, which I initially encountered on my bike, but seemed to be creeping into my daily life. Several times I found myself struggling to focus my eyes at work. Reading the packaging of my gabapentine tablets, there is the possibility that these issues might have been side-effects of this latest drug but, then again, the list of potential side-effects included pretty much every medical condition I could think of.

It was five weeks post-diagnosis, coinciding with some early season, sunny weather, that I reached something of a breaking point. I needed to escape and get back on my bike. I rode out to a nearby lake to meet some of the riders from my club. The route afforded amazing views across Bristol, with hot air balloons in a clear blue sky. It was a beautiful evening and was as good as it gets.

As I cycled back home, the fog around my leg muscles suddenly seemed to dissipate. It had been lingering there for weeks but disappeared in barely a matter of seconds. I can pinpoint the exact moment it happened; the sensation almost boosted me forwards as if muscles that had forgotten how to work kicked back in. Goodness knows the neurological reason for this dramatic change, or an apt word for my reaction - maybe "elated" or "exhilarated" - but I had a spurt of excited adrenalin that would keep me awake that night. For the first time since diagnosis I felt good again, as if something inside me had been unlocked and was working anew.

I was wary the next day and careful not to overdo it but I began to think that, if that was the end of the bout, I had coped.

48 hours later, of course, I woke up and the pins and needles were back more ferociously that ever. My whole legs felt dead again. If I was still trying to work out a new, fledging relationship with my MS, this now felt very much like a fight. And the opening bell had just been rung.

In the opening scenes of the film Batman Begins, Bruce Wayne is in a muddy jail and is being confronted by an increasing number of 'bad guys' that he has been locked up with. He battles to fight them off until the prison guards drag him away, "for protection."

Furiously kicking out at his captors, he growls, "I don't need protection."

"Not for you," a guard replies. "For them."

I want MS to regret being locked up with me.

I resolved to get back into the routine of a daily cycle to work and, with each push of my pedals, I envisaged forcing my MS away, down and out through my feet. Each movement of my legs would represent another blow landed.

On the first day of this new regime, when I arrived at work, I felt too pumped up with frustration to stop, the short fight of a 30-minute cycle hadn't even touched the sides. Instead I carried on through the town centre and sped up a local hill called Clarken Combe. There my legs did begin to burn and give way, but I carried on pushing, and wheezing, to the top. At the summit, my heart and lungs were bursting. I may have felt both euphoric and very bad, but certainly no mid-point compromise between the two. Maybe it equated to a bloodied, but victorious, pub-brawler the moment the police cars roll up.

My legs felt no worse for the rest of the day and neither did the issue with my eyes. My natural urge was to go out and fight MS again so, after work, I rode up Clarken Combe a second time and, with a tailwind behind me, it was probably the fastest hill climb I've ever done.

Since diagnosis, I had been looking for a way of dealing with my MS. This felt like it.

MS, you're going to regret being locked up with me. For the rest of your life.

One of the first things I did when I first got back from the hospital was to buy Roy Swank's "MS Diet Book". This will be familiar to many MS patients and a bible analogy seems an apt one, as its devotees are almost religious with their fervour, as are its detractors.

Swank writes (ed), "It is difficult for people who have been active all their lives to slow down. To have been driven all one's life by some poorly understood mechanism in one's body, and then be asked to cut the speed by a half or two thirds is asking a great deal. At times the patient is like an automobile with less than one gallon of gasoline in the tank. He or she can travel fast for but a few miles, then stutter and stop. Pace yourself. Don't rush. Listen to your body and very carefully monitor and control your desires."

As his book went on to describe some of the issues of MS, especially the early symptoms, I began to feel as though it had been written personally just for me.

This is a new world for me and I know that I will need to learn... and to adapt.

Maybe fighting MS is like having a fist-fight with the sea. I have always liked the urban myth about the Geordie dock worker who, to prove his toughness, used to try and brawl with 200 tonne frigates as they rolled down the launching ramp into the waves.

It sounds like there are days when I need to lie in wait and pretend to be swaying on the ropes so I can better beat my foe tomorrow. Pulling back from what I do, I've always done, is not going to be easy for me.

First long ride post MS diagnosis

Now several weeks since diagnosis, my symptoms are still there. Every morning I wake up thinking that they'll have gone but my legs still feel like two foreign attachments appended to my body. They're both numb and tingling at the same time. Some points have no feeling at all, others smart with hypersensitivity. My feet are swollen with pins and needles and I feel tired. But, although I may feel exhausted on the one hand, I also burn with a furious energy to fight my MS on the other.

The next weekend I enter a 200km bike ride: the LVIS audax.

(The term "audax" was initially adopted by French cyclists as they set non-competitive, often endurance, challenges for other riders to aspire to. Whole associations of long-distance cyclists ("audaxers") now enter such events either en masse on a given day or self-supported along pre-set routes within published time constraints. The world of audaxing is now so established that there are league tables, awards, trophies and a wide variety of spin-off competitions which seem to make this non-competitive world, as competitive as possible. The ethos, though, remains one of participation rather than speed, camaraderie rather than one-upmanship.)

The LVIS 200km audax

Saturday morning 6.30am. My alarm goes off and it's decision-time regarding the day's ride. I sit up and feel achy. Outside, the wind howls and I can hear the rain lashing against my bedroom window. The whole house is still asleep.

I can feel my MS throbbing in my feet.

An hour and a half later, I roll across the start-line of the LVIS Bristol 200km audax.

Like most audaxes, the community hall at the start was dominated by slightly wizened looking cyclists, who were bleary eyed and drinking coffee against the backdrop of an early morning murmur of conversation. The rain had abated slightly but it was still terrifically windy. I was hoping that if I could get started and get my legs warmed up, the hollow feeling in my feet would disappear. I felt most unsure of what I was letting myself in for, but I found a couple of guys from my cycle club who I could ride with – which was hugely cheering – and soon we were cycling up through Ashton Court Park with its view of Bristol. I began to think that everything would be OK.

At that stage I'd no idea no far I'd get, or how my body would hold up, but I found that I could still pedal. The first hill made me feel a bit giddy as my heart rate picked up but, there was no doubt about it, I could still cycle.

A huge tailwind billowed me north, along flat country lanes, to the day's first checkpoint (such events typically have two or three such stops where coffee and food are provided by volunteers and fundraisers).

The conditions were hard (for everyone): fierce winds and wet roads. I hid within our little group, sheltering behind other riders, head buried in my waterproof; but no one was complaining. Despite the weather, cycling is, after all, what cyclists do. I had studied the route beforehand to identify places where I could abandon if I had to: an hour later we'd be cycling within a couple of miles of my home, so my plan was to at least get there and see how I was feeling. No one was being forced to be there and certainly no one would have noticed if I disappeared off home.

The next (archetypal) checkpoint was at Doynton Village Hall. I was half-minded to ride straight past as I had the growing sensation that stepping off the bike would be painful on my pins and needles, but I needed food. As feared, I didn't feel great as I parked up and tucked into some soup – my legs were buzzing and felt alien – but I was growing in confidence that I could carry on. I committed to riding past my home and heading further south to Chew Valley Lake.

An hour or so later, the rain was calming down and the route headed up and over the Mendips. A sharp descent on the far side brought my little group of cyclists to Glastonbury. By then I was tiring, but with a growing buzz of happiness, albeit one that went hand-in-hand with a sense of anxiety. I could sense some early warning signs creeping in - my vision was getting blurred and I was beginning to struggle with my body temperature. I didn't know where all this was going but had to acknowledge the dawning realisation that it was going to be a tough last part of the ride. It was getting late too and I didn't want to be cycling in the dark with blurring headlights if my vision was going to be an issue.

As I started back to Bristol, my mood was good. I had some company and was enjoying our chat at a steady pace, but I was also getting nervous: the last thing I wanted was an emergency pick-up the first time I'd been back out on my bike. My mind was made up and, at the first opportunity, I cut short the route and made a bee-line back to the car park at the start. By then, my vision was giving me all sorts of distortions: the sensation was as though I had sweat running into my eyes, but my brow was dry. I clipped a deep pothole that I thought I was missing. My bike wobbled and I dreaded the thought of getting a puncture.

I began to sense the danger of every passing car more acutely and I wanted to get off the roads.

In the end, although the last 20km were painfully slow, running on empty, I did them. Did it. Could still do it. After my illicit short-cut, I'll never be so relieved to have registered a "DNF" (did not finish) on an event.

Afterwards I sat in my car looking at my pale face in the mirror. This diagnosis was going to change my life. I stared at my own eyes wondering what was going on behind that I could not see. That no one can see.

On the way home, I ate a packet of cashew nuts.

I felt tired and wondered what my future held.

Crunching the numbers

Multiple Sclerosis activity has been described to me as a series of peaks (which are bad) called "relapses"; then troughs (which are good) called "recoveries". The difficulty is no one, doctor nor scientist, can predict the height of any peak, nor depth of any trough; their durations, nor the gap between them. The kicker is that the troughs often do not wholly return you back to your starting point but to a new, worse-off position each time. Relapses are bad short-term, but also bad long-term. This is why the condition is called "degenerative". MS-sufferers risk always looking anxiously over their shoulder, fearing the next peak. There are a variety of MS types, but most are of this relapsing, then recovering, type.

What sufferers are keen to avoid is primary, or progressive, MS. Here there are few or no recoveries and the relapses are more frequent and more severe.

Two months post-diagnosis and my symptoms of earlier this year do seem to have settled down a bit but I really hope that this isn't yet my new "normal". I want a fuller recovery, not least because it would be my first so would allay fears of a more primary-type condition. Apparently, recoveries can take up to a year to occur so, yet again, all I can do now is wait.

I've spoken (again) to the MS nurse who has advised me to slowly increase my doses of gabapentine because I still have pretty continuous pins and needles in my fingers and toes. These make walking or standing for any period of time really uncomfortable. I still have that hypersensitivity and numbness, the two unwanted extremes, in both thighs, abdomen and, less so, on my shins. I have intermittent pins and needs in my left hand and some more personal issues regarding my water-out functions that require careful attention. I realise that this last symptom should be a goldmine for humour but I fear that I may now be past that: last week, I needed the loo eight times on a single, four hour bike ride and then five times during a single night's sleep (and, *yes, I was counting*)... it's an embarrassing disaster waiting to happen.

Last week, I was out on my bike and I started timing how often I needed to stop and wee. It was about every 40 minutes. In fact, it was so reliable that I thought I'd trick the symptom and stop in anticipation but the tactic failed. I wondered what weird twist on the "normal" my body would come up with next and what unrecognisable form I was morphing into that I didn't recognise.

However, it is still my vision issues that are the most handicapping... and worrying. My vision continues to get distorted through a series of factors which I'm trying to better understand. Certain types of tiredness seem to be the main driver and, problematically for my hobby, being out on a bike for an extended period seems to be a reliable cause. Elevated body temperature is a documented cause of MS vision problems, it's called "Uhthoff's Syndrome", and my MS nurse is adamant that this is the case with me, but I remain sceptical that this reconciles to my experiences. I'm more convinced that cycling on bumpy stretches of road (which entail a lot of head-joggling and therefore eye movement) are a key contributor. On two rides this week, descending fast on uneven roads was a definite, and almost immediate, cause. I'm now going to experiment with descending hills even more slowly than I do already - luckily, my days of fast down-hilling are long behind me anyway. Whatever other theories I might have, I have been trying to stick to the advice given to me by my MS nurse: to keep my heart rate "out of the red" and to rest periodically during exercise.

There is also the new symptom of worry to contend with. At the moment, I'm all too aware that every twinge in muscle or twitch of nerves might be announcing the arrival new MS activity. One morning this week, I woke up with pins and needles down my right arm for the first time. Although these disappeared within minutes, a few alarm bells had sounded.

Reading various MS discussion boards, I realise that MS can, and might still get much, much worse than this. There is actually quite a lot of anger on these boards directed at sufferers of "MS-lite" who complain of their symptoms whilst running marathons *(inspiring)* or riding bikes. Personally, I want my MS to be as "MS-lite" as possible. I cross my fingers, I just need to remember not to do so too obsessively to the detriment of my actual life.

My assigned MS nurse has been valuably reassuring and I have been hugely grateful for her support but everyone I speak to is very reluctant to give you any opinions on the likely progression of the condition.

“No one knows.”

"I know it's hard but please be patient."

This feels like a game we're having to play because I know, as well as them, that there is a large element of not wanting to scare the newly diagnosed. The unspoken truth is that the worst possible case is very bad indeed. So, I turned to the internet for some better data.

Predictably, figures differ, but for a man of my age, newly diagnosed, there appears to be roughly a 15% chance of having a condition at the primary/progressive end of the spectrum. No time for sugar-coating here, this basically means that you could well end up being in a wheel chair in three to five years.

If you dodge this bullet, roughly 65% of sufferers “require walking aids” within 10-15 years. If you get through this zone of progression, patients' odds begin to align more and more with non-sufferers. For example, over 20-25 years the probability of an MS patient dying of cancer is very similar (well, similar enough) to the rest of the population. If you have MS, your life expectancy is shortened by roughly seven years.

I also read that of MS sufferers who suffer visual distortions, roughly 3% experience total vision loss at some point during their lives.

I feel as though I need to know these figures – to unveil my hidden enemy – but I also realise that this is just the tip of the iceberg. It all still feels very new and I need to find out more.... to draw MS out into the honest open where we can now do battle.

As I research the above, I decide that I can wait for my NHS consultant's appointment no longer.

I make a few phone calls and book a private medical appointment with a neurological consultant from Southmead Hospital, Bristol.

£300 to seek answers to the rest of my life.

If life's a party, please can I change the music?

Three months post-diagnosis and, at last, a consultant's appointment (albeit an expensive private one).

A patient walks into the doctors.

"Tell it to me straight, Doc," he says. "No sugar-coating."

The doctor proceeds to tell him the grave seriousness of his condition.

Struggling to digest this latest news, the patient laments, "What I meant was: 'convince me you're going to tell the truth, but then just tell me what I want to hear...'"

"THE TRUTH?" Jack Nicholson barks, "YOU CAN'T HANDLE THE TRUTH!"

This week (and it felt so long overdue), I had my first appointment with a neurological consultant. We talked about where I am and what my next steps should be.

We discussed my symptoms and he explained the results of my MRI scans.

A lesion (or scar) on the brain or spinal cord, coupled with MS symptoms, would be enough to trigger an MS diagnosis. Scars on the spinal cord, as opposed to the brain, tend ("tend", but not always) to be warning signs of a more aggressive form of the condition. Their number, and size, are (very) rough barometers of the extent to which the condition has taken hold.

I could be seen to have several lesions on my brain and several more on my spinal cord. Having seen the scans though, I realised why the consultant was reticent to describe this as an exact science: they looked like an explosion in a white paint factory. My suspicion is that no two radiographers would come up with the exact same figure. In fact, it seems that no areas of the MS condition are black and white but these lesions, coupled with my symptoms, are certainly not great news. In fact, according to the consultant, this seems to be enough to categorise my condition as being at the more aggressive end of the MS spectrum.

A lumbar-puncture of my spinal fluid (which wasn't actually as bad as it sounds, nor as others had reported) confirmed what the MRI scans had shown. A bit of me had been holding out hope that perhaps I'd been misdiagnosed but this had not been the case.

So, the conversation quickly moved on to the next steps, drug decisions and new chemical names: Lemtrada; Tysabri; or Tecfidera? Blood transfusions and time off work. The benefits of stronger drugs would need to be weighed up against their stronger side effects, some so strong they could kill you, some so strong that their initial doses change your immune system for good. I was handed a pile of leaflets to read and I started typing these new drug names into internet search engines.

My consultant's advice was to get started on a drug program as soon as possible - the sooner the better - but then followed that up with the news that my next follow-up appointment, drug decision and, eventually, prescription, would not be for at least another month. These extra days might just be drips in time, but I know they'll be frustrating hours and minutes that will grate against my impatience to get started.

Ultimately, the drugs that I'm likely to start taking did not exist eight years ago. A decade ago, the odds of ending up in a wheelchair would have been more stacked against me. Now? I might still be heading there. Whatever drugs I end up taking, they need to do their work.

I asked the consultant what else I could do.

He paused for a while and gave me a considered response. "I advise that you try as hard as you can to be happy. Do not let your condition run your life."

And cycling?

"Happiness, you'll find, is the best medicine of them all."

I arrived and left my appointment in my cycling gear, having ridden from work, but I also had to pigeon-step in and out of the hospital as I struggled with that most basic of functions.

On my commute home I suffered a rear wheel puncture.

"How annoying," I thought.

Acceptance?

Reactions to a diagnosis (in my case of MS) are widely described in literature as following similar patterns to a bereavement:
Shock, perhaps confusion or denial;
Anger;
But then acceptance.

One of the several emotional conversations I have had over the last few weeks was with a fellow patient who had symptoms extremely similar to mine. He was the same age, almost to the day, as me and was even of similar appearance, slightly spookily so. He had been diagnosed earlier than me, by some three years.

Over the last few months, triggered by symptoms very similar to what I had been experiencing, he had stopped full-time work and "retired" from his sport (where he had reached a decent level). He now used a walking-aid when his symptoms were at their worst.
He was quite incredibly calm and phlegmatic about these concessions (or, at least, described himself this way). I tried to articulate the amount of fight I still felt I had but he was philosophical about this as well. His story was that he had been "furiously angry" for two or three years after his initial diagnosis - I think he had taken out a lot of that anger playing ice hockey which was perhaps why he'd got so good at it (!) - and his marriage had slowly fallen apart, but he believed that he was now calmer and happier. He described himself as growing into his condition – living with it, rather than fighting against it.

I have still not accepted the changes that MS is bringing, and will bring, to my life. It seriously agitates me. I imagine that, given time, these feelings will calm down and I too will reach my own acceptance of sorts. But I also wonder if this is really what I want – or exactly the thing that I want to fight.

As I re-assess my cycling, there are different levels of concern. Firstly, there is **immediate tolerance**: can I keep cycling through whatever symptoms I'm suffering? Secondly, there is the worry of **long-term damage:** is being out on my bike worsening my long-term prognosis in any way?

Immediate tolerance is something I can probably answer for myself. I can either cope with it, or I can't. My current symptoms of foot and leg pain I'm assured are not going to be exacerbated by exercise (when I say, "I'm assured", I haven't actually been "assured", this is just what I've been told), but, at the moment, the flow of being out on my bike is the ***only*** thing that I've found which takes my mind off these incessant pins and needles. The absence of any leg strength is depressing and exhausting but I've resolved that whenever I come to a hill I'm just going to have to use my bike's smallest gears and ascend at walking pace, ignoring commuters, young and old, as they slowly overtake. Harder to cope with are my vision issues and MS-related exhaustion, which arise suddenly and without warning. These not only stop me on my bike, but also seem to wipe me out for days afterwards with all the impacts on family and professional life.

Long term damage is harder to resolve. I'm just going to keep on asking the questions of the experts, doctors and anyone who knows more than me. Is cycling-related fatigue just being tired? Or is it worsening my long-term chances? A day in bed is worth it for a weekend of cycling but an increased likelihood of disability is not. I understand that you need rest to recover from illness, but how deep into the "red" can you go? A fast 30-minute sprint, or a slow 12-hour touring ride? Or neither? And, wrapping around this whole issue, is the psychological benefit of being happy and whether this alone can offset any other physical stresses?

I don't think I'm yet ready to concede what has been my passion for over 20 years.

My love of cycling is a love of being free; a love of being outdoors and of long descents and of tailwind speed. But it is also a love of the battle, the challenge, the hair-pinning climbs and the horizontal rain, the coffee-stop when I was too tired to carry on and the sudden view of the sea after a two hour climb. Should these things stop now?

If some elements of coming to terms with an MS diagnosis can be compared to a bereavement - perhaps a selfish mourning for a lost future that you now need to change? - I feel as though I've absorbed all this change with surprising ease, however, I do have my suspicions that I've just failed to realise it at all. There have been too many small incidents which have triggered disproportionate emotional responses.

What am I ready to give up? And what can I cling on to?

Chapter Two: The science

What is MS?

I am discovering that the causes, symptoms and prognoses for MS sufferers are difficult to sum up succinctly. I have a health issue which is unique to me and that I'm going to have to live with for the rest of my (hopefully long) life.

The exact path the condition takes would seem to lie in the lap of the Gods. There is currently no known cure so, whilst it would be extremely dangerous to ignore, advice focuses instead on not letting it run your life. Its development can be managed with diet and a variety of disease-modifying drugs and it seems that every combination of the two has its own devotees and detractors.

In fact, for the first 48 hours post-diagnosis, I was told so many times that it “might not be that bad”, that I started to wonder what all the fuss was about. I found myself having to google “what’s bad about having MS?” The answer is that it’s a deteriorating neurological condition that only gets worse and rarely gets better. Signals to and from your brain are at risk of getting increasingly fuzzy, to the extent that you may have issues controlling the feeling and control in areas of your body. At one end of the scale, these might be pins and needles in your hands and toes, but the possibilities run right through the whole spectrum, through bladder and sexual dysfunction, to blurred vision, muscular weakness and severe fatigue, vertigo and imbalance, blindness and the inability to walk. Accelerated brain shrinkage conjures up a horrible picture and I’ve been introduced to terms like brain fog, ataxia and cognitive confusion. I read that MS sufferers typically have immune systems which struggle to switch off after periods of activation (e.g. when you're ill or infected) so apparent symptoms of illness linger, sometimes for many weeks at a time.

At my age, 65% of MS patients require walking aids within 10-15 years of diagnosis.

So, although it "*might not be that bad*" – given that my initial suspicions were that I might have a trapped nerve in my back – MS is certainly not great news.

My background to MS

So, I'm now officially an MS sufferer.

A few months ago, I didn't even know what MS was.

My first two questions were, "Is that bad news?" (I'm afraid so) and "Can I still race my bike this weekend?" (yes).

I asked, "Am I going to die early?" (hopefully not) and "Am I going to be disabled?" (again, hopefully not), "Can I still cycle?" (yes, to an extent) and "Can I still go to work?" (hopefully so). It could be very bad; could be not-so-bad...

It would be easy to focus on the moment of diagnosis – the "big reveal" – and announce this as "when my world changed" but, for me, everything had already been slowly changing, for many months previously, probably for several years, as my condition morphed into a more recognisable form. In fact, I saw my own "big reveal" more as being more of a recognition of issues that I was already suffering and, as such, it felt like a vindication that could be met with relief rather than despair.

It is difficult to pinpoint an exact beginning, but I believe that I had been suffering from various medical ailments that I can now attribute to a maturing MS for seven or eight years. Being given a medical diagnosis helped to clarify many of my own suspicions and thus put into place a missing part of my own identity. Almost immediately, my own personal jigsaw seemed to make more sense.

A sense of relief came from getting an answer to a long unsolved puzzle, full of clues, red herrings, false dawns and anxieties. Suddenly, my many trips to the doctor with unexplained ailments had been justified: the bouts of intense exhaustion; the listlessness; an inability to overcome minor viruses; the repeated days off work; and the blurred vision.

What weird health oddity my body would spring next had become a running joke with my wife: I had sat for eye-tests which reported me to have 20:20 vision despite the fact that I couldn't focus on anything; I had periods of terrible muscle aches that felt like a hangover from the Glandular Fever I had suffered in my teens; winter-based depressions that I could only assume to be some sort of Seasonal Adjustment Disorder ("SAD"}; and the symptom of urgently needing the loo with only seconds notice, which had led to yet another unwanted (and embarrassing) doctor's visit. I had several blood tests all of which suggested that I was in perfect health. I had always been a sociable drinker of alcohol but my hangovers were starting to get worse and worse. Ultimately, I had decided to stop drinking entirely because even a single unit of alcohol was rendering me bed-ridden the next day, sometimes the next two.

Somewhat out of desperation, I had started keeping a sickness diary in an effort to find some sort of link between these bouts of malaise but, despite an apparently recurring seasonal pattern, I couldn't identify any obvious cause. For the four years pre-diagnosis, this diary now shows that I suffered five bouts of extended illness/exhaustion lasting several weeks each time. The worst two bouts lasted almost two months each. These were periods when I could work, but only just. I needed to sleep, (sleep and sleep) but just couldn't fight off a lassitude that I struggled to describe to my doctors.

I had begun to feel like a slightly unhinged hypochondriac but, now I'm a diagnosed MS sufferer, I have been armed with a justification for making all this fuss. I wish I could go back four years in time and explain all this to my original doctor as he kept sighing at my insistence that neither stress nor anxiety were the cause.

Where did my MS come from?

Multiple Sclerosis has no known cure, although, with recent advances in stem-cell technologies, fingers remain crossed, and experts still debate the best approaches to its treatment and prevention. Each patient seems to experience the condition differently ("my MS") with different symptoms and impacts upon their lives. No one can say how quickly a given individual's condition will progress and the variation in future prognoses pretty much covers the entire spectrum of possible health outcomes. The different types of MS are not black and white but a swirling mix of overlapping and blurry greys. Even with the benefit of hindsight it is difficult to accurately chart how an individual's condition has progressed because the identifiers of the condition (multiple scleroses on the brain and spinal cord) may remain stable as a patient's symptomatic presentations evolve and change, or vice versa. Despite all this, the causes of MS are better understood than is common belief, it's just that they are difficult to describe succinctly because they are a blend of genetic, behavioural and environmental probability factors. The condition is as difficult to prevent as it would be to deliberately contract.

Different MS patients have different variants of the condition, caused by different factors. Triggers or indicators of the condition have been computed using pools of data but no scientist has ever (or ever will!) sit down and carefully analyse where my own, individual and unique condition has come from. To tackle this frustration, I can but hypothesise:

MS is most commonly diagnosed in adults in their thirties (tick for me); but with a 3:1 ratio weighted towards women. I read (and then wish I hadn't) that men, for some reason, tend to suffer from more aggressive forms of the condition.

There is a genetic predisposition to the condition that appears to be triggered, not by a single gene, but by the complex interaction between around 100 different genes, each of which, individually, only has a small effect. If you have a first-degree relative (sibling or parent) with MS, you are 20-40 times more likely to have the condition yourself. As far as I know, no one in my family has ever been diagnosed with MS before me (*what a trailblazer!*) This is not uncommon though: only 25% of individuals with MS have a genetic disposition to the condition. I can probably assume that I sit with the majority of sufferers who have developed their conditions due to environmental or behavioural drivers instead.

"Environmental and behavioural" factors do not necessarily mean factors within an individual's control. Some certainly are: diet, tobacco smoking, stress levels and a lack of exposure to the sun to name a few, but I refrain from self-blame – more statistically significant triggers can be put down more to simple bad luck (for example, exposure to a certain virus et cetera).

Never having smoked, and (largely) having had a healthy diet with lots of outdoors sports & sunshine, I would not have said that I stood out as a high-risk individual. I do, however, read with more interest the theory that the consumption of cow's milk from an early age may later cause your immune systems to attack the myelin sheaths around your brain/spine, mistaking its proteins to those previously identified as being foreign within that milk. I wonder if all those years of voraciously eating bowls of milky cereals and iced milk drinks accidently trained my body to attack the wrong proteins? There are numerous one-off studies and publications examining (and usually falling short of anything more than apparent correlation) such hypotheses but of more universal acceptance is that MS-issues only arise if your immune system manages to start getting direct access to layers of your brain/spine that are usually locked safely away behind "the blood brain barrier". This may happen for several reasons, perhaps just bad luck, but most likely through viral infection or trauma.

In my time, I've managed to bump my body (read: brain/spine) in a whole host of different ways, most pertinently from bike, skiing, footballing and (occasional) car crashes, but it is the statistical link between the Epstein-Barr-Virus ("EBV") and MS which seem to ring more true in my case. I endured Glandular Fever (which is caused by the EBV) in my late-teens and my case was fairly typical: I was initially ill for a few months but suffered several more minor relapses for several years afterwards. When I began to start suffering from MS some 12 years later, I initially could only articulate my symptoms as being "exactly like the glandular fever I used to have" – lethargy; fatigue; aching & buzzing muscles and swollen & painful glands. To now read of a link between EBV and MS seems to completely justify what I had been saying to doctors for several years: that it felt like I had glandular fever again. Blood tests could only confirm that, yes, I did still have the virus in my system. As I tried to articulate my mystery symptoms, I found myself describing my spine as being ill or infected in some way. I had have some sympathy with the doctors who thought that I was a hypochondriac and a bit nuts.

I am not sure what I can conclude from the above: drinking lots of cows' milk, then having glandular fever, will not have guaranteed my development of fully-blown MS. On the one hand, those theories that explain MS as a disease of diet and lifestyle choices don't seem to fit (and I don't think that this is just a defensive reaction to perceived victim blaming), but, on the other, I think a simple explanation of "bad luck" shies away from an answer. It's the sort of response I got used to hearing from doctors and it translates as "we simply don't know yet." Perhaps I'm failing to acknowledge the surplus amounts of refined carbohydrates, sweetened drinks and red meat (read ice-creams, shakes, burgers, energy drinks and flavoured milks) that I ploughed my way through in my teens and twenties? I was always so active that I perhaps mistook a low body mass index and fat count to mean a healthy diet? Maybe I mistook the hours I spent playing outdoors in the summer to mean a Vitamin D rich lifestyle when, being brought up in London, I'll have spent many winter weekends hiding from the rain in cinemas and playing computer games? Appearances can be deceptive and I believe that both my doctors and I were lulled into thinking that I couldn't possibly have anything seriously wrong with me because I was doing so much healthy exercise.

Of course, who cares now? I'm not sure why but the answer to that rhetorical question is "me". It's somehow comforting to know how I have been put together and to understand that I haven't just been afflicted by the tap of a magic wand.

On this third rock from the sun, spinning through the vastness of space, our little lives all come down to atoms, molecules, blood-brain-barriers and lymphocytes. I wonder what's going on now as somewhere behind the scenes, my immune system goes about its busy work, hopefully doing more good than harm.

MS and Seasonality

Over the last couple of years there has been the welcome sight of several high-profile news releases regarding the optimistic results of Stem Cell MS trials and some of the reported results do indeed appear quite remarkable. An episode of the BBC's Panorama brought these to the attention of a much wider audience and increased awareness of the condition (albeit focussing on the more severe end of the spectrum): *http://www.bbc.co.uk/programmes/b06ss17g*

This BBC program elicited a number of, slightly premature, congratulatory emails to me from well-meaning friends but it was a much smaller 2015 study that more caught my attention: an investigation into the seasonality of MS relapses and their potential link to melatonin levels in the body: *http://www.scientificamerican.com/article/melatonin-linked-to-seasonal-relapses-of-multiple-sclerosis/*

As I struggled for years to get a diagnosis of my condition, one of the consolations I now have is a detailed list of when I suffered "relapses", and how long they lasted. These dates show quite an amazing pattern.

I list below the dates that I had been bedbound (or too ill to work) by (admittedly self-diagnosed) MS symptoms over the last five years.

Firstly, in March:

- 16th March to 20th March
- 18th March to 30th March
- 10th March to 23rd March

- 22nd March to 28th March
- 19th March to 23rd March

Then in October:

- 22nd October to 27th October
- 8th, 9th, 14th, 18th, 19th October
- 13th October to 19th October
- 14th October to 20th October

I do believe that there is something temporal that is driving these patterns. I've read several different theories about possible causations which range from a change in temperature, to daylight hours and their association with Vitamin D levels, to, more indirectly, the emergence of a new season's set of bugs and germs.

I have shared these thoughts with my neurological consultant but it seems that modern science can't yet identify the physical/chemical/neurological markers that are causing these bouts and so can't yet take the steps to modify or reduce them (let alone cure them).

The frustration is that I can almost predict the onset of a relapse. You don't need to search for long to find message-boards and patient forums that offer anecdotal reports in the same vein as mine. These complaints may vary in the detail but are united in their frustrations.

A little bit more web-surfing and it becomes clear that the vagaries of such eye-witness accounts are backed up by more scientific studies:

from Buenos Aires

https://www.ncbi.nlm.nih.gov/pmc/articles/PMC4570563/

to Rome

http://bmcneurol.biomedcentral.com/articles/10.1186/1471-2377-10-105

via Melbourne

https://www.ncbi.nlm.nih.gov/pubmed/25283272

The majority of the reports that I have found have taken statistical approaches, however, the first of the links above offers a decidedly more molecular explanation. My reaction is that such cold, hard science (although less accessible to the layman reader like me) seems to further beg the question why a better solution hasn't been found given this apparent granularity of understanding.

My summary of the situation would seem to be that the links and causations of seasonal correlation are still only hypotheses rather than findings: be they links to Vitamin D deficiencies; melatonin levels; diurnal temperature ranges; changing seasons; or even air pollution levels. As a result, NHS patient-advice has had to remain woolly: take Vitamin C and D supplements; rest; avoid stress and germs; and eat healthily. Arguably, do what you should be doing all the time anyway.

It seems to me that the most reliable solution would be to up sticks and move to a more tropical clime; whatever the reasons/causations, incidence and relapses are markedly reduced the lower the latitude you live at.

For now, all I can do is wish for summer... secretly wondering what the cycling is like in Belize.

Footnote 1: Interesting to read the following extract from Roy Swank's book on Multiple Sclerosis: "Marked changes in the temperature will be followed within a week by deepening fatigue and weakness in many patients. For this reason, in the north temperate zone, we see many patients in October and again in

April-May who complain of fatigue and weakness. The symptoms last 2-4 weeks then disappear."

Footnote 2: Remarkably, Australian researchers showed that peak MS relapse rates are indeed statistically most likely to occur in the Northern Hemisphere's earlysSpring and they even gave an exact date: 7th March (looks like I'm a week or two late!) A remarkable set of data though. Their consensus is that this is linked to a patient's Vitamin D levels (which correlate to sunlight exposure), although scientists are aware that "reverse causalities" may be at play here: a new set of seasonal bugs & illnesses (which can trigger relapses) might just be driving patients indoors, which would lower their Vitamin D readings but only as a secondary indicator (rather than as the cause). Interestingly, the same research suggests that October is the least likely time of year for MS relapses which clearly goes very much against the dates that I have recorded above. Fascinating stuff though.

Footnote 3: I add thispost-script on the 13th day of the following October. I'm just spending my sixth day of the month sick in bed, buzzing with pins and needles, exhaustion and muscle ache. The predictability of this bout makes it no more bearable. I wonder if patients and scientists of the future may re-read these accounts and be amazed at our naivety once the true cause has been discovered.

March: The Pre-and the post-truth

Pre-truth

I type this on the eve of March.

As the "danger month" approaches, I've again started pottering around the internet in search of hints, hope and (any) advice.

It probably goes without saying that I hope my March this year is better but I do have a genuine optimism that this will be the case *(the danger of hope)*:

Twice since Christmas, I've contracted minor colds but, unlike the familiar pattern of yesteryears, these have not developed into two or three weeks of MS fatigue and illness but, instead, have passed after just a few days.

I've been encouraged enough to break my own golden rule and enter a March bike race: the rather intimidatingly named "Chippenham Hilly" (it's hilly and quite near Chippenham).

I am currently suffering a mild bout of optical neuritis and the wobbling sea-sickness that this entails but, this last weekend, I cycled 270 miles, so I can't complain of MS-related weakness on the bike.

I've even fitted my posh, (overpriced), race wheels to my posh, (overpriced), race bike. I even oiled the chain... my bike, at least, is good to go, aiming to hit March head-on rather than trying to sneak round the sides.

I type the above as a statement of "pre-truth" so I can't be accused of writing with hindsight. I hope my next paragraph, "post-truth", is a glorious confirmation of my hopes. It feels as though I'm betting quite a lot of morale on this one.

Post-truth

The month of March started with my MS grumbling away. I started getting tiresome pins and needles – especially at night – and was struggling to focus on my work, specifically on the screen that I was meant to be working on. I am starting to take the symptom of blurred vision as a lead indicator of an irritated MS.

Quite how much of this was in my head is difficult to say but, because for several years I have had health issues in March, I must be forgiven for watching the month like a hawk. Although the saying goes that "a watched pot never boils", for me, this seems to rather miss the fact that if you're watching a pot carefully, you can see every little change in the water's surface and can better monitor every little ripple for a potential simmer.

Trying to unravel whether my March-malaises are just indirect symptoms of a wider anxiety is certainly something that I'm open to, but this is a process that I wouldn't know how to start.

On 6th March, I did ride in that aforementioned local bike race, the "Chippenham Hilly". The headline news was that I finished and afterwards felt a nice euphoric glow of vaguely-competitive endorphins rather than the blurred vision vertigo I had feared.

The fact that I finished 28th, I must face, is of no interest to anyone except for myself. I'm going to have to consign it to my own personal memory bin (alongside that time I holed out a 7-iron in 2008; or when I scored a first-time volley for Cockfosters FC under-16s at somepoint in the previous century). Never to be mentioned in polite company again.

Then March started to take its usual turn.

Over the next fortnight I had five days off work.

I moped about complaining of vertigo and incessant tiredness and towed my same old line about my vision "not feeling right".

I started going to bed earlier and earlier and having more broken nights' sleep with cold sores and buzzing legs.

I read that the average bout of optical neuritis lasts about one month. I know, like that watched pot, there's no benefit in fretting – I should just get on with life as best I can - but that's not necessarily human nature. This is perhaps best evidenced by a recent exchange with my ten year old:

Like many youngsters these days, my young son has an obsession with his game-console to the extent that we, like many parents, impose screen-free hours/days/weeks as appropriate.

Being told he couldn't play for another hour, every five minutes he kept asking, "Is it time yet?"

My response was that each time he asked I'd add another five minutes to his wait.

After a reasonable pause, he countered with, "I'm not asking how long it has been.... I just want you to know that I haven't forgotten...."

Such is the way with my optical neuritis. I ignore it, but wilfully so.

After about eight days, as historically seems to have been the case, I felt as though this latest bout of malaise was beginning to fade, but its last residues were still fairly suffocating. Over one weekend of family socialising I thrice had to interrupt mealtimes to lie flat on wooden floors, overwhelmed by vertigo.

I still seemed to have little, or much reduced, control over my left foot – which seemed to curl up on its own accord – and I felt weak and tired, stuck in some sort of permanent post-viral fog.

Last Sunday afternoon, the last of the month, I fell deeply asleep in a cinema, with all my plans for an active week of holiday ahead feeling like a folly. The dark tendrils of resignation seemed to be spreading. That evening though, a big turning point for me was when a dose of "Prochlorperazine" (my new anti-vertigo drug) dramatically arrested a bad bout of dizziness. I went from lying, prone on the floor and pulsing with exhaustion, to robot dancing with my son. It made up my mind that I would get back on the bike the next day, albeit armed with a bag of drugs.

My plan was, as April arrived, to immediately start riding my bike to excess.

Cycling with MS: a 900-mile week

"CyclingWithMS": of course, "cycling" and "MS" are not the only things in my life, but, for this one week in cold April, they certainly dominated. And, in their different ways, they certainly dished out the highs and lows in extremis.

Only April, but it feels like I've already seen a few false dawns this year. That said, I do believe that this last week, which I took as holiday off work, did represent a real turning point. It felt as though the balance of the scales were shifting and, at last, I was taking the fight to MS again rather than just absorbing its blows.

Monday started with me rolling my bike out of my in-laws' front drive, into the pouring rain and wind of Storm Katie.

To say that my legs felt empty would be an understatement. I didn't have enough strength to push the pedals to get me out of their drive (which is quite some hill) so I walked my bike, slowly, to the top.

As I rolled down the hill on the far side, I was acutely aware that my balance wasn't all that it should be and that the roads were hellish slippery.

This was no good, and a recipe for a crash, so I took some more of my new prochlorperazine drug and carried on very slowly.

I was having an issue with my left foot which seemed to be particularly weak and fuzzy. My solution was to put all my effort into my right leg and, once I had built up sufficient momentum, I'd then allow my left leg to join in smoother circles of rotation. I did worry that this would cause issues further down the road but decided that I'd just have to deal with those if they arose.

I rolled downhill towards Swansea Bay and approached the sea. No one else was around at 7am on an Easter Monday. It was a glorious, deserted windswept seascape. I began to think then that the day would be OK. I was determined to make it so.

By Tuesday, the ball was rolling and I was growing in confidence that I could manage the vertigo with drugs. Although the symptoms of exhaustion and weakness were harder to gauge, I was very much minded to carry on, albeit at a very careful pace. Tuesday's test was the cold. It started near freezing. I rode over the exposed Severn Bridge with a friend of mine (with him doing the towing), through two inches of hailstones. I'd already despatched my morning's prochlorperazine tablet so the bout of vertigo that hit me as we arrived in Wales was a true concern. I think the biting cold was a big factor but I don't think my friend realised quite how close I was to having to lie down in an icy puddle as we discussed the route. I was surprised how articulate my voice still sounded as I swirled with confusion. I, somewhat illicitly, took another prochlorperazine and five minutes later things seem to settle. Of course, I then immediately got a puncture on the next descent, which had to be changed with cold, fumbling, wet fingers.

Those were tough moments and as close as I got to calling the whole week off.

Some more over-the-counter medication got me to Cardiff – past the enormous Tata Steel Plant that had been so much in the news that week – and, one jacket potato and beans later, the day seemed to have stabilised. I felt really weak – and never more than a sugar cube of energy away from sleep - but slowly I was beginniing to have fun.

It was a tailwind home.

On both Wednesday and Thursday, I rode too, through two brutal, headwind hailstorms, but also under blue skies and sun.

By then, I was beginning to feel on top of any vertigo, so my focus slowly shifted to the next limiting factor – where lop-sided cycling was emerging as next biggest problem.

Cycling for miles (upon mile) only using one leg was inevitably going to have repercussions. Untangling where MS stopped and where muscular imbalance started was both impossible (and pointless) but my left foot was continuing to curl and cramp and I was beginning to get worsening tendonitis in my left achilles and knee[1].

I carried on riding at the same slow pace – along country lanes, up very gentle hills – not yet able to manage a climb of any gradient.

I carried on taking drugs. My energy levels ebbed and flowed – several times I had to pull them back from those dark caves where tired cyclists go to give up.

By Friday, I felt strength returning and the only thing that was then going to get in my way was worsening pain. I grew concerned about what lasting damage I might be doing to my left leg – such overuse of a confused limb would probably be having all sorts of knock-on issues with tendons, ligaments and bone. My back was getting achy and my left knee had progressed from discomfort to sharp pain. Despite this, my primary emotion was one of growing elation as I could feel the balance of power shifting:

I'd started the week under the thumb of MS but it felt as though I had now prised that thumb away and, with huge effort,

---

[1] *If, as a cyclist, you're ever wondering whether you can ride without full power in your left foot, the answer would appear to be yes – but with a 15% power penalty. (For the record, on my very own "CyclingWithMS" scale, the figure for severe vertigo would seem to be about 75%...)*

was now reversing those roles. It felt as though I'd broken the back of this bout and I was winning again.

That Friday felt like a proper watershed; it was only then that I realised quite how deep I'd dug those last few days and felt the welling up of exhausted tears.

That night I caught up with an old friend. I can't pretend that I felt great but our evening of socialising passed with no lying on floors and no risk of fainting. My blood sugar felt seriously low but, by now, that was more due to cycling than to MS. I slept in fits and starts but was invigorated to wake up to sunshine the next morning.

On Saturday, I cycled from London to Bristol, ready to ride again on Sunday. The culmination of my week was to be another 200km audax. Last time out, I'd had to abandon with worsening issues with my vision. It had been a violently windy day and my focus had been largely on surviving unscathed (see "*First long ride post MS diagnosis*"). This time, the sun shone and the wind barely whispered. My strength remained steadfast and I felt happy. I caught up with old cycling friends and made new ones. The rain that had been forecast did not precipitate.

I rode 250km and could have done more.

Seven days previously I had been lying in the foetal position on the kitchen floor, feeling nauseous with vertigo if I even tried to lift my head. Seven days on and I had cycled almost 900 miles.

The advice to MS patients experiencing “relapses” or “MS fatigue” seems to be to take things as easily as possible. Rest. Sleep.

I quote below from the NHS MS advice I was handed upon diagnosis:

“Periods of fatigue may develop quickly, and apparently without cause, and last for days and weeks, but rarely longer. During

these periods, patients are generally weak and may find it difficult to get out of bed or do simple chores. These spells of exhaustion usually lift or disappear suddenly, leaving only the underlying persistent fatigue."

"The only effective treatment of fatigue in Multiple Sclerosis is rest, ideally by lying down. Rest by sitting is less helpful. If the fatigue is severe, go to bed for several days. When a patient overexerts frequently or for long periods, and fails to allow sufficient time for recovery, deep fatigue may be prolonged."

These advices seem only to partially tally with my experiences. I can only go with what my body does / has done and my experiences of these debilitating relapses are that, after a week or so of being bedbound, I can then get back to real-life, albeit at a greatly reduced pace. I grimace badly for another three or four days but things do seem to continue to go in the right direction whether I then continue to rest or not.

I hope that all my efforts of this week do not take a long-term toll... but, for now, *MS, there's no way you're taking this round. I hard-earned this week – it's mine and feels deservedly so.* I just hope that, in trying to win this battle, I haven't lost sight of the war.

Certainly, the last week or so has been hugely buoying, but one irony is not lost on me:

As I rode my bike last week, I was going to bed earlier and earlier.

And my legs were still feeling fatigued and shaky.

And, as it took a while for the adrenalin of those rides to wear off, I still wasn't sleeping brilliantly.

Maybe "good cycling" and "bad MS" are not so removed, just dictated by the eye of their beholder.

Chapter Three: The six months post-diagnosis.

Fighting MS with a bike

The "Heart of England" 300km audax

A couple of months post-diagnosis and I am still trying to work out what my diagnosis means for me, what I can and can't do and the extent to which my love of cycling might need to change.

Each new week seems to bring new MS-highs and lows as I learn more about my condition and my reaction to it. This week has been no different and my symptoms – pins and needles, hypersensitivity and numbness from the waist down – have not changed.

It is the issues I'm having with my vision that continue to be the most worrying. Whenever I'm out on my bike for any prolonged period of time, I cease being able to focus. The problem then worsens until I have to abandon wherever I'm going. If I'm not going to let MS get the better of me, I need to better understand what triggers this and how best to avoid it: it feels like I need to get back to the drawing board. I've developed an approach of research on the internet; test on my bike; assess; then revisit. This whole process has actually proved quite a welcome distraction from life.

As mentioned above, my medical advice was that a rising body temperature might be the culprit so, going against years of "training" as a cyclist, I've started to set off on my longer ride with a self-imposed heart rate limit. I allow myself neither efforts nor sprints and try to keep a relaxed easy pace throughout. Last week, I started off on the south coast in Poole and although, initially, I felt great on the bike, by the time I arrived home many hours later, it had all got a bit concerning. After a few of hours of gentle riding, at about the 100km mark, my eyes had started to get confused and, from that point on, the ride had got slower and slower until, ultimately, it had become quite scary. In fact, I had become so slow that it had started to get dark which had further exacerbated the issue. I tried to shake away the blurriness but my brain was playing tricks on me. By the time I got home it was late. I was tired and relieved to have made it in one piece.

My symptom of optical neuritis is difficult to describe because it is not strictly double vision, rather it's a delay whenever my eyes demand a change in focus. This delay is barely perceptible - perhaps milliseconds - but it's enough for my eyes to be continuously flitting subconsciously back and forth as my brain falls out of sync. The effect is almost dizzying and a sort of travel sickness descends. The rapid head movements that a bike ride entail worsen the issue. Initially, I find that I can "reset" my eyes by halting for a few minutes but, when the neuritis takes a proper hold, nothing seems to clear the fog.

This week, focussing, if you'll pardon the pun, on my optical neuritis has been a mindful distraction from my higher level concerns about the MS condition. I had found the effort of trying to digest so much highly emotive new information all at once fairly exhausting. I was awaking in the night, suddenly panicking about some unknown that I had to investigate and understand. On a couple of occasions, I couldn’t get back to sleep and, instead, mulled everything over and over again into the early hours.

By Friday, I was pretty pale and exhausted. That night I started another new course of gabapentine - “do not drive or operate heavy machinery” - but had also set my alarm for 4am on Saturday morning, ready to ride the Heart of England, a 300km audax out of Cirencester.

The ride started in the rain – welcome, again, to the world of audax - and I started slowly. I'd set myself two rules: firstly, to keep my heart rate under a steady 140bpm at all times; and, secondly, to stop every hour for at least a couple of minutes. The latter was the more frustrating as it meant abandoning whichever little group of companions I'd settled into but my legs felt surprisingly good on the bike. It was only when I stepped off the pedals that the dreaded pins and needles would reappear.

As the ride slowly unfurled and I started seeing signposts that were more Midlands (Daventry, Rugby and Leicester) than the South-West, an unexpected issue emerged: in a determination to stick to a new, more MS-friendly diet[2] - no dairy, no red meat and reduced saturated fats - I was struggling to find appropriate foods to eat at each food stop. The hungrier I got, the more disillusioned I became as I searched the menus at each designated cafe-stop: they were filled with delicious buttery cakes, bacon and sausage rolls, and ham and cheese baguettes that I couldn't eat. I knew, from having learned the hard way, that a ride of this length would demand sufficient fuel and I'd need to eat what I could. My day's nutrition ended up reading:

- Food stop 1: baked beans and toast
- Food stop 2: baked beans and toast
- Food stop 3: potato and baked beans
- Food stop 4: potato and baked beans

I struggled to cope in this regard and felt more and more sluggish. I'm also not going to be able to stomach another baked bean for quite some time.

Regarding the problems I've been having with my vision, the ride seemed to replicate my experiments of earlier in the week. I

[2] See the later chapter: "The fabled MS diet"

felt absolutely fine until around the 150km mark, when my eyes started to get a bit unfocussed. The next planned-stop was still another 20km away and I got there slowly, with growing concern. I told my story to a group of my fellow cyclists and one rider's wife of 30 years turned out to also have MS,

"Enjoy life while you can," he said prophetically.

Again, just as I'd found earlier in the week, a long-ish break really helped, both my vision and my resolve. Looking at the route, I knew that the end was in sight (*aherm!)* and also that I could ride the last leg as slowly as necessary; I just didn't realise that this would turn out to be very slowly indeed. Partially this was due to non-MS symptoms which I was less concerned with (saddle soreness, tired legs and body *(toughen up)* and inappropriate nutrition) but, for the last 20km, my vision issues were back and were dreadful.

I kept stopping and shaking my head. I lay down on the verge by the roadside and poured cold water over my face. There was nothing I could do; I had hit a blurry wall and completion became an exercise in survival.

I finished alone and in the dark.

The marshal at the end looked at me and said, "You look pale, son."

I felt pale too but I was pleased that I still looked young enough to be called anyone's son.

This ride had been a test but, with plans to do a 400km ride in two week's time, I had more work to do. It would be back to the drawing board... again.

The "Brevet Cymru" 400km audax

Usually, when I'm out on my bike, I'm very much there in the moment, soaking in every sight and smell and feeling every bump in the road. The turns that come and go are seen and noted, the little descents are enjoyed and little climbs cursed.

But sometimes I find myself with my mind elsewhere, deep in thought and contemplation. When I get like this, if I were stopped and asked where I'd just ridden, I wouldn't know. I would have been subconsciously following the road - up and down, left and right - but with my focus elsewhere, turning over and over some imponderable.

Who we are, what we're doing with our lives and why we're doing it.

In deepest, darkest mid-Wales, I floated out, above myself, and continued to zoom out and out. My little speck surrounded by the night, lost in the lashing rain. My little dot, legs turning and turning, moving slowly (very slowly) back towards Chepstow. I had skipped a couple of doses of gabapentine (for reasons I'll explain later) and my pins and needles were extreme. I had them all the way down from my belly to both feet, burning toes and a swollen tingling in both arms. My vision was utterly distorted.

What am I? What remained?

I thought I could ring-fence my upper chest, my neck and "me" – my consciousness. "I" was very much still there. Then my neck and shoulders started to really hurt, although not MS related, and I could only laugh. I knew I was still there, somewhere in the front of my brain, just behind my eyes. Maybe that's all you need to still be "you".

I have asked the same question of every healthcare professional I have met since diagnosis: **will cycling in any way worsen my condition? The answer has always been, "No."**

I wasn't even in pain, not "real pain". My pins and needles were just discomfort and I was actually weirdly happy. It felt like it was me against the elements, me against MS. I was being tested but felt nowhere near to being beaten.

In the run up to the ride it felt as though I was getting more in tune with my MS symptoms and how they were reacting to the drugs, primarily gabapentine, that I was taking. I was also becoming increasingly attuned to the side-effects which felt as though they were getting more noticeable. I was getting more aware of how spaced out and tired I would feel after taking a dose so, with this is mind, I had dropped the midday dose (the middle of three) and instead was enjoying the drug sending me to sleep at night.

The previous week, I had ridden to work every day with no reported issues with my eyes or vision. The Wednesday had not been a good MS day but the rest of the week was much better. At times on Wednesday I was struggling to walk – really fatigued, muscles stiff and pins & needles in my feet – but I didn't want to tell too many people, or to moan, because that Saturday I was planning to cycle the Brevet Cymru 400km.

The route stretched from Chepstow in South-east Wales, all the way across the principality to the sea... and then back again. My alarm was set for 4am. The forecast was, as usual, for heavy rain.

Audaxers start in all their finery - shiny cycling gear and high-spirited banter; back-pockets full of food and bodies full of energy - but fast-forward a couple of hours and I felt like a bedraggled mess. I had stopped at the roadside, desperately trying to put on my second pair of gloves with fingers that were too cold to move. I had stopped being able to change the gears on my bike because I'd lost feeling in my left hand. My windproof jacket was akin to holding a tissue to the rain and I was completely soaked through. I had already had to stop four times to go to the toilet, losing whoever it was I had been riding with.

I had 320km further to go.

But, if this first chapter of the ride was a freezing cold struggle, the second chapter was a much more uplifting tale of camaraderie. Two fellow cyclists from my club took me under their wing and the roads started to pass much more easily. We chatted often, mostly not, but now I had a wheel to follow and progress felt efficient. One positive side-effect of the continuous rain and body shivers was that my body was certainly not overheating. My vision was unimpeded and I only felt first felt the twinges of blurry distortion over 100 miles in.

The furthest point of the route was the seaside town of New Quay with its steaming fish and chip shop. As we reluctantly left its warmth to get back on the road we guessed at the time – having not checked it for half a day I guessed at 5.30 but it was already gone 8pm. With time flying to this extent I must have been having fun.

The third chapter of the ride was all battle. After patches of brightness during the afternoon, the rain had truly set in: firstly, a misty, almost pleasantly cooling version; then drizzle; then, with a furious kick at the end, a torrential downpour that brought mud and leaves gushing down onto the asphalt.

I followed red taillights through the blackness, up and down, as the road surface chopped and changed. Visibility was too bad to see any folds in the tarmac, they were just announced by a new pattern of vibrations and a rattle of fittings.

Eventually I accepted that my pins and needles were getting too much and I took the gabapentine tablet that I'd been delaying. I still had over 100km to ride so I was nervous as to how drowsy it would make me feel. It was six hours past my bedtime and I knew that I needed sleep. The drug, the darkness and the late-hour all added up to a spaced-out feeling of other worldliness where I kept catching my thoughts as they drifted away from my conscious reach. "Stay Awake, Stay Awake," I repeated over and over again.

I was badly underdressed, I was soaking wet and I was shivering but, underneath it all, my core (me) felt strangely fine. I would even say that I was happy.

At 4am our group of three stopped in a little lay-by, ducking our heads to the heavy rain. My friend explained to me:

"'Type 1' fun is just fun. Pure and simple.

'Type 2' fun' is not good at the time, but when you look back on it, you realise how much fun you were having."

"And Type 3?"

"Type 3 is just not fun at all."

I eventually finished at 6am. Exactly 24 hours after I started.

That was certainly another test. Without my chance encounter with the two other riders from my club I doubt I'd have made it through.

I also felt badly ill equipped and will now go out and buy a waterproof that actually works. Ditto a more expensive front light.

In keeping with my MS diet, the list of foods I ate was a long one:

3 malt loaves
3 sets of baked beans with various accoutrements
1 vegetarian cooked breakfast
3 bananas
5 coffees
3 cans of coke
1 packet of jelly babies
5 homemade flapjacks
1 bowl of porridge
2 bowls of soup
3 hot cross buns
some dried dates
and 1 packet of sliced chicken.

I weighed myself after the ride: 73kg. Six weeks ago I was 78. I am not sure what this means for who I was and who I am now? I wondered whether the MS deep inside me had been growing or shrinking during this time.

Playing Poirot

The inexplicable is usually caused by a paucity of evidence combined with ineffective deduction.

The appearance of one, be-suited office worker on the canteen floor would, at first glance, have appeared to be both remarkable and beyond reason. Initial diagnosis of the situation will have been further complicated by the gentleman's relaxed demeanour – his apparent clarity of thought and relaxed and steady heart rate gave no clue as to his immediate past.

But there is always a trail, which can be traced to a cause, to give us understanding of the present. This trail just needs to be found, then patiently followed back in order to establish the facts.

The previous night, it seems, the same gentleman had outstayed his normal bedtime. According to his wife, his routine had been swayed by the appeals of a new TV box-set. This instance might perhaps not be noteworthy in itself but was apparently then followed by a fitful night's sleep. The cause of this, when carefully attended to, also ceases to be a mystery, for it can be apportioned to an excessive use of a new central heating system. Small temperature differences in the night have oft been reported to cause minor flare ups of neurological confusion to individuals predisposed to suffer such.

The wife's evidence further bolsters this thread of supposition as she reports that the gentleman awoke that next morning complaining of numbness in his lower limbs.

We must shift now the environs of our case to "Featureless Office Block 1" where, that next morning, I have been informed by one of reliable repute, the same gentleman emerged from his post-commute shower with red and "smarting" legs. The less inquisitive may cast this grain of evidence away but my little grey cells collate such pearls of wisdom because it is these very such grains that together create the circumstance that we later receive.

The last known sighting of the gentleman appears to have been at circa 10am when a colleague recalls him complaining of a light headedness which our patient had sought to arrest with a strong coffee.

Thus, my equation nears completion: overtiredness plus overheating, plus a bad night's sleep, plus the early signs of neurological confusion. Our gentleman clearly removed himself from his busy office environment, in retreat to the quiet confines of the canteen, where some sort of vertigo seems to have overcome him and brought him to the floor. Eye witnesses report that he appears to have dozed quite happy for almost an hour with his head resting directly, if not comfortably, on the hard-wearing carpet tiles thereof.

This, my friends, is no mystery.

Just another unremarkable day.

The huge great big, red neon light flashing above our patient's head perhaps offers the greatest clue – the capitalisation is not my own: "JUST TRYING TO KEEP GOING, DESPITE MS. SOMETIMES IT'S HARD".

We can concur that some sort of "MS" incident is here at play.

An abbreviation I will now google to determine exact meaning.

"CyclingWithMS", sometimes just "LearningToLiveWithMS".

Thank goodness for Summer

For me, winter has always been a season to endure: the dark, the wet and the cold.

Summer is the light at the end of the tunnel.

The seasons change, the clocks move on and, by the time that June arrives, the sun is shining, the skies are blue and my mood is lifted.

Over the last four or five years, what I know now to have been MS symptoms, have moved in time with this, almost like clockwork. As I have described above, my worst bouts always seem to coincide with the dark months – typically peaking in March and October.

Of course, now I have a diagnosis, these bouts can now be seen to have represented a tangible ailment – MS – and it was with this in mind that I had my second appointment with a neurological consultant last week. The last time I saw him, I could barely walk into his room. I was depressed, ill with MS and rundown after weeks and weeks of suffering interrupted nights' sleep. This time, I cycled to the appointment in good health and he described to me the various treatment options that were available to me. He handed me more pamphlets to read and I wrote down (again) the drug names I had to google (again).... Lemtrada, Tysabri and Tecfidera.

I may have had some residual pins and needles in my toes and fingers and some slight numbness and hypersensitivity in my legs – but I felt good to go.

I was back to riding my bike almost every day. Some days I'd feel better than others but, on balance, I could say that felt like a cyclist again. I hadn't had any issues with my vision for five weeks and had felt emboldened enough to take the next step and enter a couple of appropriately low-level bike races:

50 miles

Firstly, I rode in my club's annual 50-mile Time Trial. My headline should read "Great News, absolutely no issues with my vision" and this should be the only news that matters, but, somehow I find myself a bit disappointed by how slowly I rode (*I'm not sure how I've so lost sight of what actually matters?!).* In itself, this disappointment must be a sure sign that I'm feeling much better.

Steady miles ridden this year proved no substitute for actual training: I clocked 2hr 18min, albeit on a hilly course. I think I was probably one of the only riders on a standard road bike but I came rock-bottom-last in my category, miles behind guys with their horizontal aero-bars, time-trial bikes and posh pointy helmets and skin-suits. I must take satisfaction with the fact that I had even ridden the 50 - I remind myself that non-cyclists would probably baulk at riding this far, let alone racing it! My limiting factors were typical for a cyclist, rather than an MS-sufferer - leg cramps, a sore back and shoulders and tiredness - better these than vision-distortion, disconnection with my legs or an inability to move my fingers.

25 miles

Only a few days later, I then rode in my club's 25-mile event. The sunny conditions felt fast despite a strong crosswind. On my way round, I seemed to feel weirdly overweight (despite the issues I've been having keeping weight on), wheezy and unfit. The event from a few days earlier still seemed to be a weight in my legs but I got my head down, did what I could.... and took over two minutes off my PB despite the lumpy route.

No one cares nor notices my times apart from me – but I was pleased despite, again, being nearer last than to first. My vision went a bit blurry in the car park afterwards but, there I was, with MS, still very much alive. Still out on my bike.

Cyclist 1; MS 0.

A good day.

Yes, summer is when things are at their best. This year, I enjoy it all the more as I steel myself for the drug-decisions, then the treatment options, that lie ahead.

A nadir. Then a high

Four months post-diagnosis:

Nadir: Def: the lowest or deepest point; depths

When things are not going to plan one must always be hoping that a "nadir" has been reached: by definition, if this is the case, things are about to get better (or strictly, I guess, end completely which, of course, is less desirable...)

Of course, a characteristic of life is that personal nadirs are only identifiable with hindsight. At the time, there is always the risk that things are just going to get even worse.

During these early stages of my MS I've tried to continue to cycle, continue, in the most part, to work and continue to live family life. As a barometer of my refusal to let MS knock me off my course, I'm still contemplating (although admittedly with increasing uncertainty) the Paris-Brest-Paris bike ride in August this year. The last qualifying event for this was a 600km audax starting from Manchester last weekend. You would have thought this 36-hour bike ride would be the subject of the nadir in the title - my body would be getting pushed to an extreme, I'd lose a night's sleep, my muscles would be exhausted and the issues I'd been experiencing with my vision would be tested - but, no, my lowest point had come on the Tuesday, a few days earlier. This was the first time I thought that maybe MS was going to beat me and it was a moment that made me realise that whatever drug choices lie ahead of me, I couldn't underestimate the impacts of this condition. I was going to have to throw whatever I could at it.

The Tuesday hadn't been a good day from the start. For no apparent reason, my MS symptoms – muscle ache, pins and needles and bladder control – had not been good. I discussed my low mood with my wife just before my boys arrived back from school and she suggested that I take refuge in a cinema to avoid the stresses of the evening. As I sat watching a film on the big screen, the aches in my leg muscles seem to grow in intensity until they were positively pulsing with exhaustion. Sitting down didn't seem to give relief enough, I had to lie down but my legs still ached with a need to relax even more. I retreated into some sort of foetal position as my legs yelled with extreme fatigue. The film went on – bangs and explosions in the dark – oblivious to the fact that my MS was pushing me into the ground.

I was marooned in the theatre. I couldn't seem to walk and had a sudden and immediate need to go to the loo but couldn't move. This was as I low as I'd been, helped out of the theatre by a teenager in a Cineworld uniform.

I decided then, if not already, that I had to get onto a drug treatment as soon as possible. But this was also as low as it got.

My nadir had passed.

The high: a "Pair of Kirtons" 600km audax

On the Friday night, barely a few days later, I drove up to Manchester to meet my friend, my audax companion. We slept at his in-laws. I had bad pins & needles and was feeling tired and grumpy. Through the night, I had what felt like the beginnings of a sore throat and a nasty head cold but, when I woke up on the Saturday morning, all the fog and malaise seemed to have cleared. Initially I was more puzzled than relieved but, as we set off - I didn't dare even mention it, didn't want to tempt fate – barely any pins and needles.

Over the last four or five years, I've seen previous bouts of (what I now suspect to have been) MS relapses similarly clear with dramatic suddenness for no apparent reason, one morning upon waking up.

I rode my bike all day with no urgent toilet stops, neither numb arms nor hands and no vision issues.

In fact, for the first time in almost three months I felt almost no MS symptoms at all.

I chatted amiably with my friend throughout. The sun was bright in the sky and a tailwind blew. The countryside was a lush green and we rode until we could smell the sea.

We saw the sun set on one day, then rise on the next.

I ate a cold tin of baked beans for breakfast in the twilit foyer of an out of town supermarket.

It was my birthday.

Living the dream indeed.

The carrot... and the stick

Cycling is a beautiful, but cruel, mistress.

It makes you work for the good times and it dishes out some bad.

The Tour de France is on our screens at the moment. We all find those crashes to be spectacular and dramatic, if a bit gringe-worthy, viewing. It's easy to forget that each of these accidents threatens to extinguish an entire year's worth of training with all its hopes and dreams. A single incident, over in the click of fingers, can unravel hundreds of hours on the road.

Earlier this year, as I struggled my way around the Heart of England 300, I got talking to a rider from my club. He'd long been an "audax-er" (or long distance) enthusiast and had long held an ambition to ride the famous Paris-Brest-Paris ("PBP") event which, like the Olympics, is held every four years. As we ascended a climb together, he explained the various life-factors that had prevented his participation both four and eight years ago. This qualifying event, he felt, was his "last chance" as the timing of other qualifying rides meant that he had to finish that day. As he spoke, suddenly his legs gave way and we saw that his rear derailleur had completely sheared off his frame. After realising that the incident had also bent his bike's chain irreparably, he decided that he was going to have to get a (very) expensive taxi home.

His PBP was over. He could only smile, "So here ends my campaign."

Over the last few weeks, I've allowed my hopes to get dangerously high. The annual "Etape du Tour" event in the French Alps has homed into view and is now barely a week away.

This mountainous event has been a ride that I've targeted for several years, ramping up my training and efforts to try and get the best possible time. Four months ago, I had put in my entry, more as a pipe-dream than in expectation. Then, slowly over the last few weeks, it's been dawning on me that I might actually be able to take my place. I've felt fit and have been riding up hills on my bike.

I booked flights and accommodation. I bought race insurance ("Does this cover pre-existing medical conditions?") and I wondered what it this growing optimism might mean for me.

Then, four nights ago, I woke up with intense pins and needles along both arms. Really powerful ones. The next day I had a couple of weird bouts of vision-distortions. I started needing the loo with dramatic urgency again and the dreaded pins & needles re-appeared in my feet.

Last night I slept for 12 hours and could barely get out of bed when my alarm went.

Maybe there's an element of these symptoms being psychosomatic but it doesn't feel like it. It feels like MS is still there and does not want to let me ride the Alps. I thought the question was: should I race the Etape? But, like always, maybe it's not the answer that's the issue, it's whether or not I'm asking the right question. Maybe it should be: what on earth am I doing? And what am I trying to prove, and to whom?

On the Friday, I flew to Geneva with my heavy bike bag. I hired a car and had the exhilaration of driving up into the Alps, through Annecy, then along the valley to Chambery. The mountain tops loomed larger and larger up into the skies and I had butterflies of excitement.

I queued to collect my big event start number & welcome pack and mingled with all the other cyclists. The bright sunshine and the clear air felt different: they felt like holiday; they felt like cycling.

Yes - this was a long way just to ride a bike, but, as a cyclist, few landscapes can hold as much thrill. You feel as though you're where it all happens, the epicentre and Mecca. You can almost smell the Grand Tour.

If you can't enjoy riding a bike here, you're doing the wrong sport.

L'Etape du Tour

When (Sir) Steven Redgreave won what turned out to be his penultimate Olympic gold, the cameras caught him at the finishing line. "If ever you see me near a boat again, you have my permission to shoot me..."
Back he was, four years later, winning another Olympic gold.

The struggle can get pretty bad, even when you're winning (at least, so I've been told!)

I used to do a lot of running (I was a far better runner than I will ever be a cyclist) but my own white flag moment was not one I came back from. I was jogging the Paris marathon when an old, niggling knee injury suddenly escalated into something that felt much more urgent, probably best equated to a painful toothache. I tried to carry on but my lower back then flared up... and then my hip. I finished in pain. Several weeks later a consultant was showing me an MRI scan: my arthritis had got so bad that hairline fractures were appearing on my knee joint. I didn't have the heart to go back to that pain cave again, that was it for me. I waved a white flag and I haven't run since. I don't regret it, my body was spent.

Yesterday I cycled, or tried to cycle, the Etape du Tour in the French Alps.

As it happened, there were several bad accidents during the event as there are most years. I was not one of these fallers, in that respect things could have been so much worse, but a good headline would seem to be a text sent to my wife as I got to the bottom of the final climb:

"Struggling. MS symptoms bad, not sure I'll be able to finish. Might have to give in. I'm going safely, not to worry, but might be home late."

I need some time to digest the implications of where I went yesterday. What I know is that, although people talk about bravery and of "good heart" when cycling, one can only do what the body can take. Nothing can replace adequate preparation, training... and good health.

Pre-event concerns

As mentioned above, after a few weeks of much improved symptoms, for whatever reason, last week, my MS seemed to flare-up again. The night immediately before the Etape, not only did I have bad pins and needles but my legs kept spasm-ing, violent mule like kicks when I was half-asleep. It was if my mind was worried that they'd lost touch with that part of my body. I felt weak, I'd been sleeping for longer and longer each night without recovery and was back to getting up four or five times each night to go to the loo.

I did contemplate not starting, a "DNS" (Did Not Start), but, especially given all that fuss of getting there, I couldn't find it within myself to let that happen. To me, this would be losing to a force of MS-bad. I had been on rides this year when I had felt similarly off-colour and had emerged largely unscathed, so I wondered just how bad it could be. Despite the draining symptoms, I had a determined inner confidence that I could still do it.

The event

As a cyclist, one of the tricks is getting to know your own body, to know when you can accelerate versus when you need to hold back. On long distance events, you need to know how hard you can push and how hard you can't. The trouble is, when your body isn't feeling right, it's difficult to know what implications that should have. Should you abandon? Or just go at 90%? Or at 50%?

From the moment I slowly rolled across the start line amongst a crowd of other queuing cyclists, I didn't feel right. I tried to convince myself that this might just be the nerves of a big event, suppressed my concerns and began to get into the rhythm of a steady pace.

The first climb, the Col du Chaussy, was beautiful as the road twisted up the sheer sides of a glaciated valley but it was already getting hot in the morning sun. I was suffering that same symptom I'd had earlier in the year when I was complaining of a lack of strength in my muscles and I was being overtaken by a steady stream of riders. I knew I was breathing more heavily than I'd expect, my heart rate was higher and I was sweating more. The first descent on closed roads was still an absolute pleasure but the temperature gauge was rising.

I'd read anecdotally that hot weather and MS do not sit well together. If life in Bristol had not been a test of this, it soon became clear that this ride would be. Even early in the ride, I started ruing the fact that I had allowed no time for acclimatisation, not so much for the altitude as I struggled for breath, but for a heat that I was unused to.

As I started the second major climb of the day, the intimidating Col du Glandon, it was over 30 degrees and it was becoming apparent that my body was not going to let me have a clean run at this event. I could feel my every bit of me starting to struggle and hadn't yet covered a distance that I'd been comfortably doing two or three times a week for the last month. I eased off (and off) until it felt as though I was barely making progress at all. I started to feel completely empty with little or no leg strength. I knew then that the ride was going to disintegrate into a battle, not of fitness, but of will. I acknowledged this shift and reluctantly admitted to myself that I was going to have to steel myself for something of a battle.

Five kilometres up the climb, I pulled over onto some roadside gravel to remove a layer. That two minute break was to have repercussions as, a couple of kilometres later, I heard the cyclist's "dead man's wheeze" as air leaked from my front tyre. The cause must have been some shrapnel picked up at my stop and it seemed to deflate my spirit as well as my wheel. Such things happen but, rather than a five minute change, somehow it took me well over ten. My hands were fumbling and I didn't seem to have normal touch nor dexterity in my fingers. When I did get back on the bike, my right leg immediately cramped up, and then my left.
I tried standing on my pedals in order to shift my weight but, two minutes later, my right leg cramped up again in this new position. At that point I didn't think I'd finish.

My vision started playing MS tricks on me. I kept focussing on the wrong objects and, subconsciously, I'd start to steer towards them. A waistband of numbness appeared around my torso, a cold, tight MS hug, and I stopped being able to cycle directly up the hill, instead I tacked up in small zigzags like a sailor into the wind. I wondered if I was actually making any progress at all. Eventually, having wobbled to the top of the climb, I lay down and fell asleep. I had no thoughts for how long I might be passed out but, when I groggily came round, I saw that my GPS unit had been stationery for five minutes.

I gritted my teeth down the next descent, trying to appreciate the Alpine vistas all around, but I couldn't help obsessing about my body and what it was doing. I barely pedalled, instead I stretched, contorted and shook my legs on the move; too much pressure on my feet and my legs would shoot back into cramp. I had one more climb to do and I was going to have to steel myself for it. It was just before this last ascent to La Toussuire that I stopped and sent the rather grovelling text to my wife. That was a white flag moment of sorts for me. I'm not going to stop cycling, but - thirsty, hot, empty and in pain - this was getting too much. I don't think I'm just a Sunday cyclist who had bitten off more than he could chew, instead it was me who had been well and truly chewed up (and spat out). Cyclists go "into the red" but this was beyond red. My suspicion was that my MS had been always been lurking in the shadows, knowing that, eventually but inevitably, this time would come. I would break.

I did the final climb in pretty miserable slow motion and finished two hours later. I kept trying to remind myself how beautiful the views were but I didn't have enough left to care. I didn't feel elated when I eventually got to the finish line, I felt beaten.

I sat down in the dust immediately beyond the finish. It was time to confess that I couldn't take everything that CyclingWithMS threw at me, my appetite for more was running on empty.

That night I slept to the lullaby of my buzzing pins and needles. I woke up frequently but they sent me straight back to sleep each time.

I got up early the next morning. The weather, once again, was beautiful. I sipped a strong coffee on the patio and felt emotional. I took a deep breath and resolved to get up back on my bike.

<<Don't let MS be your excuse. It is "you" just as much as the scar on your leg, the colour of your eyes, or your love of your children. Blaming MS for something is no different from blaming yourself.>>

Thank goodness my Alpine holiday was based on a mountain summit, not at the foot of a valley.

I got back on my bike and rode downhill for 25km. I don't think I pedalled more than two or three times as I swept round the hair-pinning turns. Sun on my face, no one else around.

Another 24 hours on, I went back out and tried a climb. I rode glass-pedals and kept my heart rate at walking pace. It was a stunning, early morning in the Alps. Crisp air, blue skies and quite staggering views. The day was clearly going to be a scorcher but not yet. The day was still at its best before the high thirties of the midday sun arrived.

A driver pulled over with a friendly wave to let me overtake on the descent. The empty road had a perfectly smooth, newly laid surface and the shiny new hub on my rear wheel purred with pleasure. The air felt so fresh, clean and pure and I was so very much outdoors.

I took a tough beating on Sunday but I did love being there... and love being here. Maybe I'm just a silly ageing man who needed it: I'm embarrassed that I couldn't help myself from harking back to a previous year when I had raced the Etape as hard as I could... then rode another 50 miles back to the start to pick up my car. I need to remind myself that everyone has stories of "what they used to do"; I must cut out the melodrama, enjoy the wonderful pleasures of cycling when they are offered and keep smiling.

Remember it's all just about riding a bike.

As I've tried to continue my cycling through MS, my approach has been to battle on. If I've planned a ride, I've just gone on it. At times, this has meant cycling when very weak and, at times, cycling when probably I shouldn't have been, but it has also meant that I haven't felt beaten by this condition, not yet.

Maybe I'm not the cyclist I was but I am still trying to live the life that I want to. I'm still angry at my condition, not accepting of it, again, not yet.

I may have been broken this week but I feel that I have to keep going. I still want to be out there, riding my bike. Once more, I'll get back to the drawing board and try to work what went wrong in an effort to stop it happening again.

The drawing board (again). Cramps

A first for me this year has been the very unwanted appearance of leg cramps on my bike. This is what really killed me on the Etape when I rode over 70km with every pedal stroke driving cramp in both legs. I've suffered these cramps maybe five or six times (although never previously to this extent). Anecdotally I've heard that dehydration (more directly, electrolyte deficiencies) coupled with under-training (or over-exertion) are the primary causes so I did some internet research, which is always dangerous:

Remarkably, given all of the anecdotal conviction, there is no proven scientific link between dehydration (or mineral-deficiency) and cramps. Arguably, this is because such a complex link is very difficult to "prove", even though it probably does exist. Consensus seems to be that there are multi, varied causes for cramps but that rehydration and better training do seem to be the most reliable defences. Muscle-stretching is the best short-term, emergency cure.

Then I started reading words that set my MS alarm bells ringing: "neuromuscular fatigue" - fatigue which contributes to a breakdown in the normally efficient neuromuscular pathways that control the movement of our muscles. This rings truer to me: "Neuro" (again).

Is there a bodily function left which MS is not going to touch?

It seems that MS can affect anything, but maybe the greater risk is that I make it my scapegoat for everything.

Bounce-back-ability

I found the immediate aftermath of my MS diagnosis a fairly confusing time as I tried to make sense of what it meant for my life and for my future. It was suggested that I start writing a blog, not least to assemble all my thoughts in a therapeutic way. As I was struggling to find anything in the MS literature that tallied with my interests, hobbies and lifestyle, the title "CyclingwithMS" seemed to make sense.

Through my blog, it was heartening to receive words of support from family, friends and even interested strangers and other cyclists. One message that has been repeated is that some of the challenges I face as a cyclist should stand me in better stead for the MS hurdles that lie ahead.

I hope so.

My experiences this year have made me ponder a bit more about what resilience, or mental strength, mean. The ability to keep on (and on) without breaking in the face of an adversity, pain or challenge is certainly a strength of sorts, but I am increasingly of the belief that it is an ability to carry on after a beating – to keep going after a defeat – that will become more important for me going forwards. I'm going to have to learn to adjust strategies, to adapt and to evolve so that if one approach fails, I can take a deep breath and try another.

A colleague has just seen his son through training for the Marines. He relays that one night-hike physically broke the group. They arrived at their destination exhausted and hungry. They were given five minutes rest then told to get up and repeat.

Some dusted themselves down and set off again. Although they went quite slowly, they would have done so again and again. Others stopped right there and threw in the towel.

I know that MS is not a person, nor is it an object I can wrestle within a ring. It's a function of a mis-firing immune system which involves messages to the brain, molecules and biochemistry. It's just science, like the plankton in the sea or the atoms in the sun. Seeing it as a foe who can be beaten helps give me greater appetite to fight and creates the illusion that I can win so, for now, I persist with the mind-games.

In "The Hustler" Eddie Felson (Paul Newman) plays a titanic game of 8-ball, head-to-head against a legend of the game, Minnesota Fats.

As the frames (and hours) tick past it becomes less a battle of talent, more one of focus and of will. Perhaps the more talented player, Paul Newman, undoes his top button and begins to look more and more dishevelled, speech slurring with whiskey, whilst Minnesota Fats changes into a freshly pressed shirt, re-slickens his hair and dusts himself down, ready to go again. He was in it, not for the battle, but for the war – for that was what needed to be won.

After the Lord Mayor's show: serotonin

If ever you're wondering what's possible on a bike – and just how crazy some cyclists are – consider the friend of mine who has just completed the "Transcontinental Bike Race" from Belgium to Turkey. He did it unsupported, with the clock never stopping, sleeping under hedges and going over the Alps. He did the same last year – a massive event – and talked about, not only the tiredness afterwards, but a mental and emotional flatness, the post-Olympic low. Most people are probably familiar with this sensation immediately after a peak of adrenalin or the stress or a major event. If you've been focussing on a given moment or goal, when it's gone, normality suddenly seems a bit slow (or empty?) because you've become so attuned to being driven.

I've returned from the beautiful Alps (featuring the very un-relaxing Etape du Tour) but in cycling terms, and in CyclingWithMS terms, flatness is where I've found myself.

The week before the Alps, I'd been geeing up my MS-ing body, pretending, both to it and to myself, that cycling in the Alps would be possible. Persuasion through adrenalin and excitement got me so far but, when I rode the event, I barely crawled over the line. I think I'm still wearing the psychological and emotional cycling-scars.

I feel that I stretched on tip-toes up to an event which had been inspiring me to get out of bed every morning but, now without all that anticipation, I'm struggling to overcome the MS-lethargy that I'm suffering. Athletes and cyclists need rest and recovery (yes, I know), but I feel that this current lassitude, buzzing with pins & needles and other lower body issues, is more than just physical tiredness.

Earlier this year, I rode a succession of audax events with a possible entry to the Paris-Brest-Paris ride on my radar but, after very careful consideration and discussion with my audaxing wingman, I've decided that this would be a step too far. Despite all those efforts to qualify, I feel as though I'm treading too thin a line with my MS at the moment and I don't want to risk falling off the edge. My friend and I are going to try and do something else in its place; something that will hopefully be less nocturnal, more scenic and less crowded. It's only four years until the next one anyway...

Feels to me like I need a new source of serotonin.

My friend and I exchange emails and lists of cycling pipe-dreams. The initial lists are so far-flung as to be almost ludicrous: cycling the Nile, the Great Wall of China, across Australia and down to Cape Town. Realism, both financial and marital, eventually kicks-in and our gaze settles more on Europe. Then more on France.

I recall my recent excitement of driving up to the Etape. I remember thinking that this was the centre of it all and I remember, and regret, how badly I seemed to mess up my ride there.

Eventually we agree at an attempt to ride a derivation of La Route des Grandes Alpes, a designated, and well sign-posted route from Geneva, down south to the Med, that takes in many of the most famous Alpine climbs and cols. Flights are bought for a few weeks time; routes are planned and time booked off work.

I tell my friend about my MS, but neither of us really know what it means, so we push on.

Whatever happens (*see Chapter 5 to find out!*), at least my serotonin levels feel as though they have been topped up again.

Chapter Four:
An MS diet

The fabled MS diet

Upon diagnosis, revisiting or reappraising one's diet is a recommended first step.

There are a number of suggested "MS diets" – which range from the *"do not do anything different, just eat healthily"* to the *"cut out everything apart from fruit, veg and seeds"* – all aimed at decelerating the progression of the condition. These diets all have their devotees and their detractors and I fully acknowledge that the science behind all of them is unproven (see *http://www.nationalmssociety.org/NationalMSSociety/media/MSNationalFiles/Documents/Diet-and-Multiple-Sclerosis-Bhargava-06-26-15.pdf*), however, adopting a diet towards the less drastic end seemed to me to be a low cost, low risk approach, with potentially large benefits.

The concept of an MS diet really stems from the work of Professor Swank, whose long-term study of MS patients over a 30-year period showed remarkable health benefits associated with adopting a diet low in saturated fats (<20 grams a day). The evidence he presented seemed almost incredible at a time when there were few, if any, alternative approaches to tackling MS. Today, even though there are now numerous disease-modifying drugs available to patients, his dietary recommendations are still very relevant as they do not suffer from the potentially severe side effects of the pharmaceutical equivalents and are of low (arguably zero) financial cost.

The diet is, without doubt, healthy and, in MS-terms, some of its supporters are almost religious in their faith in it. Message boards are alive with patients convinced that the diet has nullified ("cured") their MS and they highlight numerous scientific papers which support links between MS progression and patient behaviour/diet. However, – and it's a big however – the mainstream medical community (read, in the UK, "official NHS advice") continues to shy away from a direct recommendation of the diet. The NHS's much more softly-worded advice is to pursue a Mediterranean-style diet where possible (plus Vitamin D when required). The powers-that-be are unconvinced and, given that the benefits of the diet (according to Swank) should be measured over years (and decades), no study has been able to achieve clinical proof either way.

The NHS-advice initially might appear unduly reticent but, now I'm trying to stick to this diet, I'm in no doubt that the strict discipline that it entails should not be underestimated. I have found that the diet is onerous when eating out, eating with friends or going on holiday. And the diet's instructions, at least, as per Swank, are clear: to get maximum benefit it has to be followed at all times. Any breaks set you back a disproportionate amount of time so it needs an all-or-nothing approach. I can see why the NHS guidelines retreat from afflicting MS patients with the additional pressures and stress – yet another list of things that they need to do obsessively – when there is no clear scientific evidence that the diet has any bearing on MS progression at all.

Swank's original MS diet has been refined and modified by contemporary "experts" - George Jelinek probably being the highest profile or, at least, the most visible on the internet. Focus may have moved away from exacting measurements ("science") to easier-to-follow generic advice ("art"), but the core tenets remain the same: reduce "bad" fats; increase "good" fats; and supplement with Vitamin D. Avoiding dairy products is a further, although secondary, recommendation.

With a deep breath I decided to:

- go partially vegetarian (continuing to eat low fat, white meat)
- cut-out foods containing significant amounts of saturated fats (out with chocolate, crisps, ice cream, chips and cakes)
- avoid fried food (how I'll crave that smell of morning bacon!)
- significantly reduce my consumption of dairy products (I'm going to wholly cut-out cheese which, to my dismay, will rule out future pizzas)

My main sources of saturated fat are now going to be in the form of cod liver supplements, linseed and flaxseed oils.

I enjoyed some novel tasting sessions as I sought the most palatable, low fat alternative to cows' milk. I lined up soya, rice, almond, oat and even hemp alternatives, sipping and swilling like a wine connoisseur.

When I spoke to MS nurse on the phone this week she also suggested cutting out caffeine as a way of combating bladder issues but, at that, I drew the line.

The immediate implications have been a significant increase in our food bills (by about 10%-15%) and me losing several kilos in body weight. I am 6"1 and 78kg so I did not exactly have much to lose. I'm simply finding it hard to consume enough food to keep my weight on (although this is probably great for hill climbing on my bike!)

On one hand, I seem to have absorbed my logical transition onto a new, fat-free diet quite calmly but, on the other, I suddenly felt like tears when I saw the "free ice-cream" voucher than I'd been given for Christmas. I talked to my son about a potential holiday to America, then irrationally welled up at his excitement at the thought of sharing a milkshake at an American Diner.

A cyclist's MS diet

A few weeks on the diet and my suspicion was growing that this new approach was not helping my tiredness. I may have been back on my bike but I was struggling to keep my weight on.

I was being disciplined about my new diet and was rotating my way through a set of healthy, new meals (of which I was getting increasingly bored!) These were usually some combination of white fish, pasta, salad and veg, followed by fruits and low-fat yoghurts, but I was ending up feeling hungry too much of the time. My wife would find me "snaffling", which essentially means me staring at a food cupboard or fridge, craving "a little something" to satisfy my appetite, even after I'd eaten.

Looking at the website "Strava", which I use to log my cycling miles, I can see that, on average, I ride about 40 miles a day which, very roughly, translates to burning up about 2,200 calories. This is the recommended diet for "an under-weight man looking to put on weight." To put this another way, to fuel my cycling I need to eat, not only my own recommended calorie intake, but also, in addition, the number of calories recommended for someone actively looking to put on weight. If, on one given day, I only eat a "normal" diet, the next day I need to eat three "normal" days' worth just to catch up.

I've read blogs written by hard-core ultra-marathon runners who are vegan, so I know that this approach must be possible. I will struggle to eat more volume as it already feels like I'm eating mountains of food, instead I need to find more densely-packed, high-energy intakes. It's been suggested that I go and see a dietician (*sounds pricey...*) but my suspicion is that this might just lead to a recommendation of high protein vegan food. These are well-publicised and I think I'm already aware of the benefits of beans, pulses, seeds et cetera.

Unless I start drinking flaxseed oil out of pint glasses, I feel as though I'm going to turn into a very thin broccoli (although, admittedly, it would be nice to return to having such a full head of hair...)

I don't think, however, that there's such a thing as "neuro-hunger". I stand by the opened fridge and look at another bag of spinach. And low-fat Soya Milk.

And broccoli...

Update: *Two years later, I remain steadfast in my efforts to pursue a careful diet. Although the science behind it remains debated ('debatable', even), I still feel that the diet helps me feel empowered. It feels like the one thing that I can do to actively counter my MS. Certainly when I'm within the confines of my own home, I have been able to settle into a much more comfortable routine of shopping only for what I can eat and what food types I need in order to feel well-fuelled.*

Tweaking my MS diet: science, art or unwelcome distraction?

A year later and, of the many aspects of my life that have changed since diagnosis, it is my new MS diet that I seem to have discussed the most. Everyone can relate to the concept of a new diet – and it's a good MS-related conversation piece that doesn't necessitate delving into the gory details of more personal symptoms and strife. The diet is, essentially, no more than a healthy one that anyone could (or probably should) consider because of its long-term health benefits.

Early experiences of my MS diet, predicated largely on the avoidance of all saturated fats, were that it didn't require the onerous reading of ingredient labels that I feared. Essentially, I just needed to avoid red meat, dairy and the majority of processed (aka junk) foods. This approach seemed to be working well, although I was occasionally surprised at the hidden saturated fats in some foods: some vegetarian meat-substitutes especially, but also avocados, olives and some nuts (e.g. walnuts) to name a few. Of course, these aren't "unhealthy" foods but it was revealing when I actually looked at their nutritional labels for the first time in my life.

I think that the fact that my MS diet is healthy (at least, compared to the average diet in the UK) is not really in question. Of more pertinence to me are: is it actually helping me keep my MS under control? and are the benefits, which do need to be carefully weighed up against some of the downsides, actually worth it?

My initial forays into the world of ingredient listings and saturated fat measurements felt intuitive and I was happy to do my food shopping on a common-sense basis. Now, a year later, as some of the sacrifices of social and eating pleasures start to weigh heavier and there are no obvious, visible results to talk of, I've been feeling the need for this to be bolstered by something more palpable (statistical or concrete) if I'm going to continue to subject myself to such self-restraint.

I recall too an early scene from the TV series, "Breaking Bad". If you're not familiar with it, a chemistry teacher, Walter, ends up in cahoots with a small-time local drug dealer, Gretchen, to illicitly manufacture ("cook") the drug, crystal meths. Their early exchanges somehow paraphrase my thoughts above, regarding the cold, calculating power of scientific accuracy:

Gretchen: *This ain't chemistry – this is art. Cooking is art. And the drug I cook is the bomb, so don't be telling me.*

Walter: *The shit you cook is shit. I saw your set-up. Ridiculous. You and I will not make garbage. We will produce a chemically pure and stable product that performs as advertised*

Walter: *I don't know. Just...doesn't it seem like...something's missing?*

Gretchen: *What about the soul?*

Walter: *The soul? There's nothing but chemistry here.*

Using exactly calculated chemical measurements Walter then goes on to create the purest and best crystal meths that Gretchen has ever known.

Molecules, atoms and their reactions are not magic, neither are the body's processes; they are chemistry, with known reactions between specific quantities of known chemicals. If art is the finessing of the output, the real-deal is in the numbers. I was increasingly aware that I had no hold on what my numbers actually were.

If I may weave in another reference to popular culture, in the film, "The Martian" (or the book, if you're more high-brow), scientist Mark Watney is stranded, alone, on the planet Mars. The situation looks bleak but Mr Watney is a resourceful fella. The character, played by Matt Damon, takes a look at what scant resources he does have available – principally a few seeds and some bags of excrement – stares at his camera and announces:

"In the face of overwhelming odds, I'm left with only one option... I'm gonna have to science the shit out of this."

I've decided to take his approach. Albeit a slightly more low-brow alternative to cultivating a Martian potato farm.

After all, the geek shall inherit the earth.

My assessment

For three days, I wrote down everything I ate and drank. Using ingredient listings, I added up totals for my intake of unsaturated fats, saturated fats and calories.

I was surprised how low my calorie intakes were. Given the volume of food I ate, I *only* consumed 2,600 and 2,800 calories on the two days (which is only slightly above the recommended average). To my naive surprise, much of the bulky food I was eating had little or no calorific value. For example, a large dinner of vegetables, pasta, a very large salad and a stir-fry recorded negligible amounts.

Swank recommended less than 20 grams of saturated fat a day. Note that Jelinek adjusts this to nearer 30 as Swank omitted the cumulative impact of saturated fats in good foods (e.g. even a slice of whole-wheat bread or glass of soya milk contain some saturated fats which add up over a day). My average figures were 17g of saturated fat and 42g of unsaturated fat (for which Swank gives no recommended figure). *Note that these numbers excluded the five tablespoonfuls of linseed oil that I added, as recommended by both Swank and Jelinek. Somewhat surprisingly these small additions contained an additional 5.5g of saturated fat and 41g of unsaturated: e.g. an additional 33% and 100% of my total daily amounts.*

Given that I'm also taking daily Vitamin D supplements and that my daily diet included eight portions of fresh fruit or veg, I'm now more confident that I'm doing what my prescribed diet intends.

But, what of the impact? The impact upon my MS is nigh on impossible to measure. Luckily though, for the purposes of my experiment, over the last few years I have had more blood tests than your average Lance Armstrong. This was largely because of the years of MS symptoms that I suffered pre-diagnosis when doctor after doctor puzzled over my symptoms and ordered blood test after blood test in order to try and work out what was wrong with me. The result is that I've got a steady record over half a decade of my cholesterol scores (HDL being "good"; LDL being "bad"). Most tellingly, I also had my bloods done just before I was diagnosed, and, again, last week, over a year of dieting later.

Pre-diet, both my HDL and LDL can be seen as being pretty steady. The recommendation is for your (good) HDL to be above 1 – my average reading was 0.85, with only one reading above 1 (i.e. it was a bit low). The advice on (bad) LDL is to be less than 3 – my average reading was 3.3, however, this was skewed by a one-off reading of 3.5. All my other readings were under 3 (i.e. pretty reasonable).

In summary, my cholesterol readings were certainly not too unhealthy but there was scope for improvement.

Last week, a year of dieting and my good was 1.2 (the highest reading I've ever had) and my bad was 3. Jumping to a conclusion, my new diet would seem to have bolstered my HDL (good) but to have had little impact on my (bad) LDL. In fact, my LDL is now the second highest its ever been which feels like something of a disappointment to me.

So what?

Last year, my MS felt out of control and I was desperately keen to do anything (everything) I could to put the brakes on.

Now, it feels more in control but I consciously remind myself that the long-term risks are still there and the potential downsides to the condition so terribly severe.

On balance, I am going to continue my strict diet, certainly for now. Longer term, I very much hope that I'll have a growing confidence to ease up on my efforts, not so much when I'm at home in my own kitchen, but principally when I'm out and about, in restaurants or at friend's houses because these are the times when I feel as though I've been giving up the most.

As a final thought, I repeat the advice offered by my neurological consultant, then later a derivation of the same by my MS nurse:

"Happiness, you'll find, is the best medicine of them all."

I just need to find a shop that stocks it. That one is definitely an art not a science.

Update: *I have now been on my MS diet for two years.*

My latest blood readings report that my good HDL is 1.3. This is the highest it has ever been.

My bad LDL is 2.1. This is significantly lower than it has ever been before.

Wider reading on the subject collaborates that the body takes time to adjust to new diets but after a year or so the body's processes and systems will have done their remarkable work of adjusting to their new circumstance. My readings would appear to support these theories.

Whey?

It's a funny old game, cycling.

Especially cycle-touring.

Trying to do something bigger, faster, more adventurous, more exciting... more new, more "more" than before.

Seeing what you can do and where you can go, seems to be an exercise in, bit by bit, identifying limiting factors, then one by one trying to overcome them.

Planning to do some high mileage adventuring this (2017) summer, my latest concerns have been calorific. The challenge has been to try and take on-board, then usefully digest, sufficient foods, all in the right proportions, to keep me running steady on my bike, rather than slowly descending down & down until I hit empty which sometimes has been the case.

The issue of appropriate food intake has been complicated as I stubbornly stick to my self-prescribed MS Diet. Having surmounted the initial hurdle of the logistics of new shopping lists, it became clear that the biggest challenge for me would be taking on enough proteins to keep me fuelled. As described above, I was too often eating bowls of delicious, fresh and nutritious salads, quorns, veg and pasta, but still craving more building blocks before I went to bed.

I strongly believe that listening to your own body as carefully as you can is the best measure of what you're eating too much, or not enough, of, but, in this regard, I haven't best worked out a way to answer my own demands.

Given all the tablets that my MS condition has necessitated, I've long eschewed any additional artificial supplements to my diet. I've been steadfast in the belief that I didn't want to consume products born more from the science labs than from the countryside... until now.

My stubbornness was ultimately broken when I listened to an interview with long-distance cyclist extraordinaire, Mark Beaumont. In amongst countless other invaluable tip-bits, he was eulogising about the power of the protein-smoothie. I have long turned to smoothies for post-ride nutrition. Off my own back, the recipe that I had devised through an unscientific approach born of trial and error, was for milk (*non-dairy!*), oats, banana, linseed and cocoa. This was as far as I'd pushed it but, in his interview, Mark was stressing the value of additional whey powder, designed to provide the extra protein that a tired body needs.

As a result, rather against my intuition, I bought myself one of those massive, industrial looking tubs of weight-lifters protein powder. The packaging even had a bodybuilder flexing his outrageously over-sized biceps on the front.

I started the course, one scoop a day plus one scoop after a hard ride, and, I can't believe I'm saying this, but I'm now a complete convert. The light-hunger that I've had so often, for so many years of cycling, has had its edge taken off.

Protein calculations (with apologies for some maths)

My cycling (hobby/habit/obsession) can roughly be described as doubling my calorie needs. Roughly 4,500 a day compared to 2,200.

Random google-searching suggests that I should therefore be doubling the associated recommendation of protein, from 60 grams ("g") up to 120g.

The most common hard-hitters, protein-wise, in your average UK diet are red meats (10g per 100g meat) but, because my MS diet has meant abandoning these, I've been turning to chicken breast (8g) and white fish (which has slightly less). Quorn equivalents are slightly less again.

A dinner-serving of each is roughly 250g so multiplies these figures by x2.5 (i.e. a helping of chicken gives you 20g protein, quorn more like 12-15g). To get these levels of protein from pulses/beans/lentils you'd be having to eat roughly 1-2 (pre-cooked) cups in a sitting which is a pretty large helping.

When I started my new diet, my main, and sometimes only, protein-boosts were at dinner. These would be roughly 20g servings (as above). My other meals would major in carbohydrates (grains, cereals, pasta or oats), salads and fruits... and lots of coffee. Even if I add in the protein from these foods, my early, very-rough calculations don't need much finessing to see that I was suffering a considerable protein-shortfall compared to my calculated 120g requirement. I was probably consuming half that figure (or less).

The introduction of two scoops of whey protein a day provides a protein-boost of 25g. Even including this, it still looks as though I'm in surfeit. I'm going to have to continue seeking out other, preferably more natural, sources to add to my diet as well.

I'm still trying to listen to you, body, whilst acknowledging that I sometimes need a nudge in a more sensible direction.

Before penning this chapter, in anticipation of the amusing header "Whey? Wye", I rode my bike over to the Wye Valley and tested my protein-filled legs on some hills.

So far so good.

When I go back in a few weeks, I wonder if my newly bulging biceps will still fit into my aero cycling tops....

The extra costs of supplementing a diet with protein can be a bit prohibitive. I did a quick run-through of my kitchen cupboards and shopping lists to calculate the cheapest gram of protein that I could buy. The results are a bit surprising because, despite all the new, fangled science behind high protein, processed foods, it's the good, old fashioned foodstuffs that would appear to win out: granary bread, milk and chicken.

(see Table 1, below, "The protein you can buy for £1")

Table 1: The protein you can buy for £1

Food Type	**Protein (g/100g)**	**Protein (gr/pack)**	**Cost (£/pack))**	**Protein (g/£)**
Granary Bread	15	122	1.00	**121.6**
Skimmed Milk	4	82	0.99	**82.6**
Frozen Chicken	25	250	4.50	**55.6**
Fresh Chicken	31	310	5.79	**53.5**
Eggs	6	89	2.00	**44.3**
Quark	12	60	1.50	**40.0**
Baked Beans	5	75	2.00	**37.6**
"Protein" Wraps	16	34	0.90	**37.3**
Tinned Tuna	26	166	5.00	**33.3**
Whey Powder	69	345	11.00	**31.4**
Skyr Yoghurt	9	41	1.40	**29.6**
Frozen Haddock	24	96	3.30	**29.1**
"Protein" Granola	13	52	2.00	**26.0**
Quorn Mince	15	44	1.79	**24.3**
Quorn Chicken	14	41	1.90	**21.8**
Quorn Sausages	9	22	2.00	**11.1**

Chapter Five: Disabled or athletic? Cycling my way to treatment

Disabled or Athletic?

The paradox I can't articulate

Last year, I was bed-ridden for 22 days. The clear majority of these were MS-related. This does not include the countless other hospital/doctor appointments and blood tests (*OK, I couldn't resist counting, the figure was nine*). I am self-employed and the main income-earner in my family so, after promptings from an internet messageboard, I started to look into what disability benefits might be available should my condition deteriorate: Disability Living Allowance ("DLA"); incapacity benefit; and Personal Independence Payments ("PIPs") all seemed to be possibilities.

Upon review, PIPs, designed to help those who require care during periods of disability or chronic illness, appeared to be the most pertinent to my position. Qualifying as being appropriately “disabled” is the first step but, to my surprise, along with cancer and AIDS, an MS diagnosis automatically qualifies you in this regard (who knows the politics behind this? Parkinson's, to give just one example, is not on the list). You then have to be assessed against a list of criteria to determine whether or not your condition qualifies you for financial help, but the very concept of this was making me feel edgy. I had visions of an undercover Panorama report sensationally revealing the fraudulent nature of my claim: “This work-shy bed-sitter missed 22 days of work last year... but also cycled almost 12,000 miles, entering bike events with reckless abandon and racing up hills across the South-West, laughing with friends and having a wail of a time.”

This strange dichotomy of my life was well illustrated over the course of five days last week. On Thursday, I was on something of a high: I was feeling as strong and fit as I had done for months. I'd just had two hugely enjoyable, fast days on my bike and was feeling an inner reserve of energy that I hadn't had since mid-summer. All my interactions were laced with tentative optimism and I had a growing belief that my decision to tackle MS head-on was already doing its good work.

But then I had a real setback when a weekend family wedding turned out to be the perfect storm for my MS: lots of standing up; a single alcoholic drink; and, as the disco started, echoing noises, lights and blurs. My neurological system just couldn't cope. A bit of light-headedness became dizziness, then nausea and a growing sense of vertigo. I went pale and became glued to my seat. Physically I could walk but my mind wouldn't seem to let me, as if I was refusing to let go of a hand rail.

After a solid night's sleep, the noises in a coffee shop the following morning were still too much for me as I seemed to lose the ability to differentiate between sounds. Background conversations were all I could hear. My family's voices became disorientating and spun my senses and my balance.

The next day though, I did feel much better.

Then, by Tuesday, only one day later, I was back to feeling 100% again.

Within a week, I had blasted my bike up one of the steepest climbs in Bristol and ridden 70 miles into a furious headwind and rain just because I wanted to.

I had also been unable to cope with the sound of conversation in a cafe and I had barely been able to put one foot in front of the other.

Does that make me "disabled"? A cyclist? Neither? Both? Or, like MS, some in-between truth lost in a hundred shades of grey.

***Footnote**: My research into a PIP claim was interesting. Although my MS automatically qualifies me as being "disabled" the number of days a year in which I require care is not sufficient for a claim, nor is my perceived immobility. Claimants have to require care for 175 days a year to qualify, only when they reach this level will the seriousness of their condition be assessed. This tick-box approach is an interesting morale debate: a claimant could be horribly disabled 174 days a year but not qualify, whereas a claimant who requires supervision the whole time, but who never exhibits any symptoms, would qualify (e.g. if you had epilepsy and might suffer a fit at any time, you could qualify if supervision was deemed necessary 365 days a year).*

I can only hope that I'm never ill enough to qualify... not least because there appears to be a perilous amount of paperwork involved in making a claim.

Pre-ride. On the brink of something *(hopefully not a precipice)*

June 2015

Sunday, a week ago, a bug hit my family. One by one, we succumbed to a 24-hour ailment which meant grumpy, pale faces and hours in bed. At the back of my mind I was a bit concerned about the potential impact on my planned holiday to the French Alps but with over a week still to recover, there was an element of relief as well.

But, by Tuesday, things were looking a bit bleaker. The progression was all too familiar to me – a minor bug slowly escalating into more and more MS symptoms. The pins and needles were worsening and my upper body exhaustion was kicking in. Come Wednesday, I was spending a third day in bed; on Thursday, I called in sick to work and could barely lift my head off my pillow. A walk downstairs to the kitchen left me pale and exhausted, lying on the lino floor. My muscles were buzzing furiously and I had no strength. I hadn't eaten a proper meal all week because of nausea. A dread was growing, my holiday getting closer… I called the friend who I was due to meet in Geneva. I was still desperately keen to get on that plane but it wasn't looking good.

The planned holiday was to cycle "La Route des Grandes Alpes", a famous cycling route from Geneva to Nice, taking in some of the world's most famous and toughest climbs. Over 500 miles in five days with almost 70,000 feet of vertical climbing. I looked at the route and contemplated contingency plans… railway shortcuts… car hires… avoiding certain summits…

The holiday had been wholly booked, and paid for, so I called my travel insurers. I would need a doctor's note if I didn't travel so, on Friday, I dragged myself to the surgery and sat, head in hands in the waiting room, with cold sweats and shakes. The doctor said I would be crazy to travel and wrote me a note for two weeks off work. I called my friend again and, on balance, he decided to cancel despite already being en route to the start.

It felt very much as though I'd badly let him down.

I talked (and talked) to my wife about the possible options. On balance, I was determined to at least get myself to Geneva. In the worst case, I could hole up by the lake for five days and drink coffee. All I had to do was to get myself to the airport on Saturday morning.

On the flight, I fell into an unconscious sleep from runway to runway and, even then, only awoke when my neighbour was preparing to disembark. I slept too for the whole three hour train journey that followed. I still couldn't stomach a proper meal but did feel a bit better after all that shut-eye.

Geneva

When I arrived in Geneva, the first step was to get myself the 20 miles to my hotel. I brought to mind the mantra shared with me by an audaxing friend: *"Bit by bit; bite-sized chunks"*.

It was raining and dark. My front light had been damaged during the journey and wasn't working so it was a slow ride despite being entirely flat. Eerie, and not to say a bit dangerous in the dark, and me feeling weak with tiredness, I arrived even later than planned and the hotel was dark. The only light was a glowing-blue goldfish bowl in reception.

I ate a bread roll for dinner, took a steroid and then a gabapentine. I had a bout of diarrhoea but didn't know if that had been caused by the drugs or my illness.

Sunday morning was meant to be Day 1 of the ride, if I was going to attempt it. When I woke up I could hear rain pattering on the shutters. The early morning view of the street was one covered with puddles.

I rolled out, feeling somewhat empty, into the dark.

50 metres later, I stopped in the warmth of a “boulangerie” for a croissant.

Another 500 metres and I pulled off the road again to put on my full rainproof gear – feet already wet through. If I was going to go for it, this was going to be one long day.

The start

Cycling into Geneva in the dawn was an other-worldly experience. Rain sprinkled down on the lake and the cobbled streets, criss-crossed with tram-tracks, glistened in the streetlights. I do love cycling through city centres as the sun comes up, a dreamlike quietness pervades and the empty lakeside bars with their overturned chairs still look hung-over from the previous night out.

I hadn’t planned this early part of my route well and found myself going back and forth down side streets and over footbridges. At one point, I had to walk down a long staircase, across a bridge, then back up more steps on the other side. The sound of my cleated bike shoes echoed in the emptiness.

Eventually I arrived at Geneva Train Station. The start.

Decision time. If I was going to abort, this was where it would make the most sense.

I bought a banana and drank some water. I had definitely improved since yesterday. Even more definitely compared to the day before. I figured on another 48 hours of feeling weak. If I could just tolerate that, I'd have the rest of the holiday to enjoy. What to do?

I contemplated my options, making my mind up first one way, then the next.

Ultimately, I turned my wheels south and starting slowly pedalling towards Annecy.

The deciding factor was the thought of MS rotting away inside me. I chose to carry on because that seemed to represent my best defence against MS, refusing to let it win.

Come to the edge, he said.
We are afraid, they said.
Come to the edge, he said.
They came to the edge, He pushed them....
and they flew.

Christopher Logue, 1969

La Route des Grandes Alpes: Part 1: A tough road

I felt as if I was on holiday when I rolled into Annecy, halfway through Day 1. A Sunday market was in full swing with all its smells (baking and crepes cooking) and vivid colours (fruit, veg and freshly cut flowers). All around the lake, mountains loomed, up into the clouds where I was intent on going.

This first day was hard. I persisted more for the days to come when my illness would hopefully have dissipated. There were pleasures along the way, especially riding alongside Lac Annecy, but these early miles were largely an effort to avoid abandonment; slow, but steady, in the misty rain. I averaged about 11mph on the flat that day rather than the 16 I'd usually cruise at.

That night, I still felt too ill to eat much dinner. On Day 2, I would be running on empty. Day 2 would also include my first real climb.

The next morning, I awoke, delighted to have had a really solid night's sleep. I did a mental checklist of body and limb and although my MS symptoms were definitely improving, I was aware that my physical weakness might become a real problem. The first few miles were a gentle pleasure but I knew that these were just the preamble to the imminent Col de la Madeleine, a 27km climb. By the time I started that ascent, it was already uncomfortably warm. I knew that it was going to be hard but I was beginning to frame this ride as me versus MS. If I could beat the ride, I could beat the condition. In my mind, it was becoming something representative, that I simply could not give up on. I tried to convince myself that the stakes were higher than they were... that I *had* to get to the top.

Empty. Hungry. Hot. I pedalled as gently as I could, at all times with the ultimate summit in mind. I fuelled myself with a fear of my condition, tapping into whatever emotional energy I could find and kept going because I was scared what capitulation might mean.

I zigzagged across the road when it got too steep. I remembered back when I was eight years old when my friend, Paul Bennett, was earnestly explaining to me how to run if you were being fired upon. "You have to keep zigzagging. And keep going. If you zigzag you can't be hit."

MS felt like a dirty great big cloud gathering behind me. I kept going.

I remembered too my first insight into mortality.

My Grandmother, who had always seemed so utterly full of life, came to visit one Christmas with a continuous and rasping cough. A few months earlier, she was full of all the energy in the world but now I was told that she was dying from cancer.

Although she seemed suddenly so weak to me, on Christmas morning she came down, dressed in her Sunday-best, ready for church. She even had her hat pin ready, a hang-over from a bygone era of immaculate appearances for special occasions and family dinners.

She had dusted herself down and was ready to carry on.

I looked down at my sleeves which were messily pulled down. My knee warmers, put on in the early morning cold, had slipped down to my ankles. One of my bottle racks was rattling loudly and needed a tighten. My rear derailleur needed adjusting. I was getting some friction from my shorts and needed to sort out some chamois cream.

I reminded myself of my own golden rule: keep on top of the small things before they grow into something too big to cope with.

I felt really weak when I stopped. I couldn't seem to undo my helmet strap which suddenly seems so fiddly in my cumbersome fingers.

I read "Into Thin Air" by Jon Krakauer, an account of tragedy on the slopes of Everest, and one particularly poignant section stays with me: Rob Hall, one of the climb leaders, had become marooned near the summit. He was trapped by his own belay, a tool he'd have unclipped from hundreds, probably thousands, of times before, but the frostbite in his fingers meant that he couldn't quite undo the fitting. Heart-breakingly his wife was still in radio contact with him and begged him to try one last time, "For me. For your children."

His fingers just wouldn't work. He never came down.

My little inconveniences were nothing and would be easily overcome.

I looked at my feet as they pedalled. I have written the initials of my two boys, one on each shoe. One turn for R, then one for A.

Having struggled for almost two hours, the realisation that I wouldn't quite make the summit came quite suddenly. My legs, just like that, had nothing more. I wobbled to a complete, exhausted standstill.

Incredibly, at that moment, I saw by the roadside my wife and two children. I couldn't believe it – "Look! There he is! There's Dad!!"

They jumped with excitement and started to jog alongside me.

My wife's hat blew off and she had to stop to get it.

Alongside Ryan, little Adam came running towards me, his little legs pumping a hundred times a minute to keep up. He gets so upset when he can't keep up with his brother I was worried that he'd cry but, when he got left behind, he was smiling and waving.

His older brother kept running longer than I thought he would. Eventually he slowed down too but he was still beaming a great, big smile.

What a moment! But, just when I thought it was over, I saw my mum and dad by the roadside. I couldn't believe it. They, too, had come all the way to France to cheer me on. My dad was waving his arms and clapping, "Go on! Go on!"

He was red in the face, but laughing...

Then I woke up.

I was in my childhood bed. I had been laughing in my sleep *(What a funny dream that had been!)*. My head was lying on my old "Danger Mouse" pillow (I wonder what had happened to that?)

Something didn't feel right though and why was my pillow covered in spiky grass?

I woke up again. This time I was lying on the roadside verge. According to my bike computer I'd been stationary for just over 10 minutes. Of course, the ghostly apparitions of my family were nowhere to be seen.

I was 10 kilometres from the summit.

Then there would then be a 20 kilometre descent.

Then 20 more kilometres, on the flat, to my hotel.

"Bite-sized chunks."

And, now, I actually felt quite well rested.

I look you in the eyes, MS, and you can see that I'm not beaten. See that you haven't even touched the sides.

La Route des Grandes Alpes: Part 2: Cycling heaven

Five days of cycling, 530 miles and, with a few wrong turns, what turned out to be over 73,000 feet of vertical climbing, all self-supported and on my own.

It should still be fresh in my mind, I only finished it a couple of days ago, but it feels like a tapestry made up of hundreds of little dots and to focus on one or two moments would be to miss the picture as a whole. This tour can only be described as the whole thing. The beginning and the end may be the clearest punctuations but it was so much more about the journey than the destination.

Fate had dictated that I was to do the whole thing solo, sometimes miles from any other human being, so I had a lot of time to think as I watched the world slowly changing in front of my wheels. I thought about my life, my family and the future & past. I cursed the weight of my panniers and wondered when the next water stop would come.

Over the latter three days, I did several climbs, a couple of hours of riding each, barely seeing another person, car or bike. It felt as though it was just me, a road and a view. Each summit, which started off looking like such a monster, would slowly get chiselled away as my bike edged skywards. Bit by bit, I was able to take them down, tapping out a rhythm on my pedals, heart beating in time. Each time it felt like I was slowly bringing to its knees a giant that towered over me in strength but that could be beaten by a gentle persistence and a thirst to see round that next bend.

The clarity of the air and of the light, air so crisp that a ripple of wind would chill your skin, but a sun that would still burn you. I'd climb the cols removing more and more layers, often finishing in an unzipped T-shirt, but would shiver at the summit as soon as I'd stopped, before I descended down the other side with full body warmers and a snood.

Regarding my bout with illness, I knew in the middle of the night after Day 2 that I was going to be OK. Having struggled to eat for five days, I woke at 3am suddenly urgently hungry. I wolfed down a plain baguette (*admittedly, a bit bland...*) and then had too much adrenalin to go back to sleep. Instead, I spent half an hour checking over my bike and gears. This is how my bouts of MS usually end, suddenly, in the night, like a switch has been clicked. I felt depleted and weak the next day but not ill. I'd broken the back of this tour and still had three days left to enjoy.

By Day 4, I was properly back. I was growing stronger and stronger as the day went on. Every little bit of food and drink seemed to replenish me more. Featuring Cols Bonnette and Vars, I did almost 5,000 metres of climbing that day, carrying my own baggage every inch of the way. I even climbed an optional extra that I hadn't planned into the route just because the fancy took me: the Col de Lombarde, which edged me across the border into Italy (*Ciao!*). After my illness, I was back to feeling capable and the world was opening up before me again.

That fourth day was possibly the best day I've ever had on a bike. It's difficult to express exactly why without just listing the superlatives that came to mind at every hair-pinning turn: the views were magnificent, with variety too, and drama. Sweeping vistas afforded sight of where I had been and of where I was going – stretching right off into the distance. There were some small sections through shrouding woodland but largely the climbs were under an expansive horizon on perfect roads. Waterfalls and white-water rapids passed me by and tree-lines were surpassed. The smaller vegetation would slowly thin out and the cols themselves would often be bald and windswept rocks. I would touch their tops before screeching down their far sides, back into the trees and their warmth.

This was some sort of cycling heaven.

Over the course of my tour, 21 cols came and went.They have already blurred a bit in my memory; another summit, another twist or turn. The Col du Bonnette probably deserves special mention. The self-proclaimed “highest paved road in Europe” certainly felt on top of the world at almost 3,000 metres. After an obligatory photo (actually the only one I took all tour), I turned down its descent and passed my first signpost to Nice, my ultimate destination. It felt then that I was very much on my way.

Each little French village was somehow more picturesque than the last. After every col, I’d seek refuge in the next settlement’s cafe and sample their espressos. They always tasted great, always strong and one never quite enough. My routine became an espresso from the cafe and two bananas from the "epicerie". I cursed the number of times I forgot the opportunity to also replenish my water bottles.

Moment by moment, the metres became kilometres and the hours became days. The Alps drew me closer to the Mediterranean and the landscape changed. The ravines grew steeper, the soils lightened in colour and the architecture shifted from A-frame chalets to thick-walled, white courtyards. The wildlife progressed from the odd, lost and startled deer, to hundreds of lizards scuttling for cover and the occasional snake slithering off the road. The air lost its crispness and the wind lost its bite. The permanent drizzle from the first half of the ride was long forgotten. A new smell appeared, of warm tree sap, sizzling in the afternoon sun.

Early on Day 5, I glimpsed my first sight of the sea, still fully 60 kilometres away.

The final descent down to the coast was so long that my hands hurt from having to brake so hard and continuously. I came down from a deserted summit to initially encounter my first car, then a small queue. I removed layer after layer of clothing as the altimeter dropped away. More cars joined more recently re-surfaced roads and the drivers started to overtake with more aggression and urgency. It felt like I was re-entering civilisation.

I reached the seafront with my T-shirt soaking wet with sweat and water bottles empty. The sun was scorching hot. The beach smelt of a thousand layers of suncream.

Although elated to have reached the sea, I still had work to do. I had to catch my flight from Nice Airport in five hours time so, somewhat in keeping with the trip, I then had to hot-tail it along the coast as fast as my tiring legs would take me. A detour through Monaco almost undid me as I became lost in a labyrinth of one-way streets and 25% climbs. My sat-nav tried to direct me up one stairwell after another, the wrong way up one-way streets and, at one point, straight into a shop’s automatic doors. I cast my mind back to the navigational issues I'd had in Geneva five days ago and it made me reflect on where I had been in between. At one point, I waited at a red light behind two red Porches and a Bugatti and missed the wilderness from whence I’d come.

I wish I’d had more time to appreciate (and to celebrate) my arrival in Nice but I had to rush to through its suburbs to catch my flight. I did make time to pause at the seafront though, as is tradition. My face was wind and sun burnt from the day’s extremes, my cold Coke tasted great. I looked at the waves gently lapping at the beach and the couple of super-yachts bobbing in the bay.

I felt incredibly... happy.

I arrived at the airport almost exactly two hours before my flight was due to leave. I drank a beer and slept on the plane – the deepest sleep of a man with a small ambition just fulfilled.

I had set off on this trip in pieces. I had felt physically wrecked, nauseous and shaky. Five days later, I felt tanned, capable and elated. Cycling was again my defence, and attack, against MS.

Me versus the condition. Cycling was coming to represent my refusal to succumb.

Everesting

It is now six months since my diagnosis and summer is drawing to a close.

Happy half-birthday, MS, hopefully many more to come.

The emotional intensity of the first few weeks has subsided into a pattern of slowly getting to know, and trying to better understand, my condition.

At its worst, MS has felt like an evil enemy, hitting below my belt with surgical precision, kicking me when I am down and adding new symptoms before I've to come to terms with the last. The couple of days when I felt as though I was losing the ability to walk were as bad as its got.

Sometimes it has felt like a dark and brooding cloud, hanging all around me, perhaps not raining but threatening a torrential downpour at any moment. It's been impossible to grasp, rein-in or control, a mean-spirited vapour.

On occasion though, it has almost felt like a faithful companion, never leaving me, always there. At times, it has been no more than the odd gentle nudge so that it is not forgotten - the ever-present pins and needles, a bit of numbness here, a bit of hypersensitivity there. These aspects have become part of me in a way that I almost don’t mind. Maybe this is some crazy Stockholm Syndrome but, on the good days, my MS is just an undercurrent of my personality that I don’t even find particularly unwelcome. It even elicits unexpected messages of support from old friends, some of whom I haven’t heard from for years. But, even during these lulls, I never forget that this companion has a dangerous temper and worry about what he might do next.

It's probably a good lesson for life: to always see the good in something bad (and, I guess, vice versa). I like the thought that **one's greatest weakness can also be a strength; but what you perceive as being a strength may actually also be your greatest flaw.**

In Chuck Palhniuk's Fight Club, Tyler (played by Brad Pitt in the film) accosts a terrified high-school drop-out and threatens him with a gun, "You are going to die, Raymond." When satisfied of his victim's fear, Tyler persuades him to return to his studies and then lets the man go: "Tomorrow will be the most beautiful day of Raymond K Hessel's entire life. His breakfast will taste better than any meal you or I have ever tasted."

After periods of illness, the moment when my MS symptoms subside always feels like the coming of a second summer. When this is the case, I not only feel good, but happy. Pins and needles in fingers and toes barely register a mild inconvenience. It makes me feel, like Raymond K Hessel, intensely free. The last month of late Indian summer has been good.

Really good in fact.

I have cycled to my in-laws in South Wales and back (twice) and I set an unexpectedly competitive hill climb time in my club's monthly competition. I have been sunburnt, the mornings have felt light and the nights short. I have been chasing my boys around our garden and the local park.

With future unknowns still hanging over me, I've made the most of this period of freedom to go out and set all the benchmarks and PBs that I can add to my, otherwise rather empty, list of cycling palmares. I've ridden 10, 25, 50 and 100-mile PBs and, pretty ambitiously, but much less successfully, a

200km one as well. These are done now and, whatever next year and beyond may hold, I can look back at them as what I once could do, "back in the good old days."

That left just one more solo event that I wanted to do: the grand-daddy of them all. An event so ridiculous that it would seem like a folly to any non-cyclist and probably as a behaviour akin to madness to most cyclists (I dread to think what a non-cycling, MS sufferer would think)... welcome to the concept of "Everesting". This is a cyclist's repeated ascent of a selected hill until the total elevation gain exceeds the world's highest peak. This is an undertaking that would stretch most athletes and one which MS would certainly do its best to prevent.

Earlier today, I ticked Everesting off my cycling bucket list. I rode 300km, up and down a single hill that runs West to East out of a small Cotswolds village called Lacock. I yo-yoed this random stretch of road, Bowden Hill, 63 times until my altimeter tipped over 8,748 metres of climbing.

I started before the sun had risen.

I watched the traffic slowly appear and intensify around the school run.

I stopped for refreshments at the pub at the top of the hill and for lunch at the pub at the bottom. Other cyclists crossed my path with friendly waves, before the sun disappeared into cloud for the afternoon and I saw the same school-run cars coming back to reverse their morning journeys.

There was a torrential downpour that dowsed the road in the early evening and the descent which had become so familiar took on a new personality with more threat and darkened menace.

As the sun set, the temperature dropped markedly and for an hour or so I thought that I might not quite make it. The hours were ticking by and I was getting desperately low on energy. Then, right near the end, a couple of my cycling friends rolled up with fresh provisions of soft drink and chocolate milk and my strength was restored.

I finished the last of the climbs only minutes before midnight and, by the time I'd descended back down to the foot of the hill, it was a new day.

I'm not sure whether this "achievement" stands as an exhibition of determination and strength or as a terrible neglect of other things in my life that should hold greater importance – not least my health. Maybe I'll wake up tomorrow with a clearer head on this one...

I reflect on the fact that my greatest weakness (MS) is certainly giving me a strength to prove it wrong; although whether this risks also becoming my greatest flaw is perhaps something I can ponder another time....

For now, I feel like a victor so, to me, the spoils of a satisfied night's sleep.

October: H-ill Season

October.

Suddenly the mornings are getting dark again. And colder.

As I commute to work, I'm now setting off in moonlight rather than daylight.

This is not my favourite month.

It is also the time of year known to Bristol's cyclists as "Hill Climbing Season". There are a series of annual hill races, short sharp sprints against the clock to round off the cycling year. They're easy events to enter: they're run "time trial" style, one rider at a time so you never get left behind; and no one really notices what times you get so there's no embarrassment necessary (although my times do their best!) I try to enter three or four of them every year, more to participate in rather than to compete, but note my wording: I say "try to enter" because October is also my own personal "ill season".

To recap (see *"MS and seasonality"*), before I had my MS diagnosis, I'd had several years of intermittent bad health. I became so frustrated that I started to keep an illness diary in an attempt to try and find rhyme or reason behind these apparently unconnected bouts of malaise. I took to highlighting periods of time when I was either off work or unable to cycle and these diaries now form damning evidence against October. I can now see that in every October for four years I missed at least five days of work through illness ("bed-bound"). Over the same time period, I had highlighted an additional 16 days when I was too ill to get on my bike ("house-bound"). For four years, I've been spending one in every two days in October either bed- or house-bound.

The fact that I log all my bike rides on the website Strava adds to this compelling evidence because I'm in the habit of labelling each entry in order to keep a record my cycling adventures *(I'll pause for a moment for you to digest this geekiness...)*

With hindsight, these titles from Octobers-past now seem to read like great big flashing MS warning lights: "Felt strangely lethargic on the bike today"; "Couldn't get much power today, legs felt numb"; "Felt tired on the bike despite 12 hours sleep"; "Felt awful today, went straight home to bed"; and, what now seems like an MS classic, "Not sure what was going on today, felt as though I was losing feeling in my legs."

Despite now having an MS diagnosis, I still don't know why my Octobers are so bad and, perhaps more pertinently, neither does modern science. March is exactly the same. My established pattern is that I'm then in relatively good health through the summer.

Anyway, back to this October and the "West DC Hill Climb Weekend" with four hill climbs to be raced over two days. With disappointing predictability, the previous week saw my eldest son ill in bed with a fever and a heavy cold. My youngest was up the night before with his own terrible cough. I woke up myself on Saturday morning feeling crap. I'd had what can only be described as remarkable night sweats and felt dizzy with the sniffles and itches of an impending bug. As sure as night follows day, I then registered two pretty slow times on that day's events, slower than my already modest times of last year.

Then, on Sunday morning, I woke up feeling great. I felt like an embarrassed hypochondriac after my concerns of the previous day but then registered two equally slow times for that day's events.

I must remember not to let MS become my excuse.

I need to remember that, some days, I should be happy to be at the start-line, still smiling, still riding, aware that no one cares how fast I go.

These last few months post-diagnosis have allowed me to reflect again on why this condition had proved so hard to identify. I've had perhaps three or four mini-bouts which echo my experiences of the last four or five years. Although they have now become more intense, with more obviously MS-like symptoms, they still seem to start in exactly the same way with a minor bug or cold escalating into an all-over-body, buzzing exhaustion that usually lasts a week or so plus. This is what my recent past has been plagued with but, historically, by the time I got to a doctor's surgery, perhaps 5-10 days later, the symptoms would be subsiding and I'd put it down to another odd virus that I'd somehow picked up. In this regard, the more serious relapse that I suffered earlier this year, which precipitated, at last, an actual diagnosis, has to be seen as being a "good thing". I can now start to confront the underlying cause and this is one thing that is different about this October.

After much reading, googling and a merry-go-round of marital conversations, it's nearly decision time regarding what disease-modifying-therapy ("DMT") I want to pursue. I have an appointment with my neuro-consultant next week with the ambition of making my choice in that regard.

If this summer risked lulling me into a false sense of security regarding my condition, October has persuaded me to reach for the biggest red button I can find.

"You're proving irritatingly difficult to kill, (Mr Bond)"

I have anthropomorphised my MS. I imagine it (him) like a pantomime comic book super-villain: dastardly and cunning; never to be trusted in his deceit; my own arch-enemy. For a while this summer, I thought I'd shaken him but now I see that he's still clinging on by his finger nails, conniving devil that he is... but, today, I smile to myself. He may think he's weathered the worst but my defences so far (a new diet plus a few steroids) will feel like mild irritants compared to the treatment-bomb that he's going to be hit with soon.

Poor him.

I've been doing my reading and have been talking to my neurological consultant, it's soon going to be time for me to wheel-in a disease-modifying-treatment ("DMT"). This is the best weapon against MS that modern science can wield. Perhaps it's even overkill – even comic book bad guys elicit pity when they're beaten.

A DMT is to be the next critical stage in my offence against MS and I've decided to apply for a course of a drug called "Lemtrada". Lemtrada's trademark name is "Campath". To my initial confusion, I found that the two terms are almost used interchangeably so must apologise if I do the same[3]. My

[3] *Probably a pertinent point to also apologise for swapping between kilometres and miles, metric and imperial, throughout the book. This has not been done entirely randomly but is designed to reflect the circumstances and locations involved. Some events (e.g. audaxes and European distances) are publicised in kilometres, others (e.g. time-trials and UK/USA distances) are in*

treatment will be starting in a few month's time, roughly seven months post-diagnosis.

My decision to go ahead had been made by balancing the drug's effectiveness against its side effects. Lemtrada, within the confines of the NHS, is probably the most nuclear of options and it is one can you can only do once, split into two separate adminstrations. It's a mild chemotherapy served cold over a week-long period, repeated a year later. It's designed to "reset" the malfunctioning elements of an auto-immune system but it's a careful balancing act. Choosing the treatment involves inviting something powerful into your system, fully in the knowledge that it can knock-out other bodily processes as well. It's not a decision to be taken lightly (and I'm not). The list of side effects is both intimidating and long. The consultant had to be convinced I was serious.

So is the title of this blog being said by me to MS or by MS to me? Maybe I just like the phrase. I hope my arch enemy doesn't have the breath to speak so many words. But, if he is reading this, he should be warned: I'm not only saying it with a smile but with a playful accent as well. I have a plan and he doesn't know it.

---

miles. To add to this confusion, I tend to record my rides in kilometres but, for some reason, I aspire to speeds in miles-per-hour. If it helps avoid controversy, one mile is equal to 1.61 kilometres.

Chapter Six:
Lemtrada Round 1

The lemtrada decision: treatment minus three months

For me, despite all the vast wealth of opinions, reports, studies, blogs and pamphlets available, my decision to go-ahead with lemtrada was largely based on the act of the drama that was a 30-minute meeting with my consultant. He was very keen that the decision be mine so I questioned (and questioned) him about the risks and the benefits before then signing-up for the chemotherapy treatment. I signed-up soberly but confident that I had tried to make the decision as dispassionately as possible, despite the subject being just about as emotive, or passionate, as they come.

Feeling, as I do now, so much better than earlier in the year, it felt a bit odd agreeing to start a course of treatment later this year. A second, slightly reduced dose, will be administered 12 months later. It will involve a week in hospital, possibly plus several weeks of illness and MS flare-ups afterwards and the very real risk of some serious side-effects but, in making the decision to go-ahead, I only had to think back to that day when I thought I was losing the ability to walk. I might be feeling good now but there's something going on in my body that I need to take action to stop.

Trying to understand, yet alone relaying, exactly how lemtrada works gets me into intellectual deep waters so probably best just to summarise its processes as a "re-booting" of the immune system. I can liken this to a return to ground-zero, like switching off a frozen laptop. When it turns back on again, the theory is that the bugs will have disappeared. The magic of the human body, or I guess of the laptop in my example above, is that the user doesn't need to understand how this fix happens, it just does, out of sight, hidden deep within the inner machinations of the body's atoms, molecules and DNA.

Because I, the patient, cannot truly get my head around the exact details of "immunity-replenishment" (I soon get lost when told that lemtrada will be attacking my lymphocytes, monocytes, some dendritic cell populations and, to a lesser degree, natural killer ("NK") cells and other leukocytes), I have had to rely on the guidance of my trusted neurological consultant, coupled with a bit of high-level, largely web-based, research. The problem is that the guidance is not black and white. The treatment has the risk of some potentially very serious side-effects. The decision to commit has to be balancing act between risk and reward, cost versus benefit. It becomes an "elective" medical procedure (e.g. one made by choice) rather than an "acute" one.

At the highest level:

The "pros" are based upon the analysis of large data-pools which show that, statistically, MS patients are likely to suffer fewer relapses post-lemtrada, and have reduced disability scores both, very roughly, by a factor of 50% (MS Society).

The "cons", again, are probability-based. The chance of thyroid dysfunction is still ~40% (MS Society); the risk of something more serious – you can't get more serious than death – are small, but not zero. Minor side-effects are much more likely, but I still take the view that, if these are short-lived, I can tolerate them as long as they're offset by long-term benefits.

The web is a dangerous place to try and research "science". I quickly happened across a blog written by a patient just starting their first course of Lemtrada: "I'm nervous because there's 1 in a 1000 chance of me dying because of this treatment" (my first reaction was that this must be an ill-informed statistic); and others which discussed the risks in more heart-felt ways: "I want to be around to see my children grow up and have children of their own. If I have to attend weddings and the births of grandchildren from a wheelchair, that is my fate. But I can't quite accept the thought of dying from my MS treatment and missing all of those things."

In summary, the most striking points from my internet trawling were:

Firstly, how unlikely you are to actually die, either directly or indirectly from lemtrada.

The results of clinical trials show that more patients died having been hit by cars, or by a train, or from motorbike accidents, than by any side-effects *(Alz. Advisory Committee Briefing Document BA103948)*. In fact, these, and other such results, did make me ponder quite how many causes of death seem to be lurking around us at every turn! That said, there were two, albeit indirect, deaths during trials which did relate to the treatment: one from secondary ITP and one from sepsis. Furthermore, ~3% of patients (again, MS Society) suffered from immune thrombocytopenia ("ITP") which can kill you if you don't treat it quickly. To put this in perspective, very roughly patients in the clinical trials suffered a similar mortality rate as mothers giving birth in India or Cambodia (to give two random examples) in 2015.

Secondly, although I knew that lemtrada was a "new" drug, I was surprised at how small these pools of statistical test-data were and how recent.

The major drug trials incorporated hundreds of patients worldwide, not thousands, and many secondary trials only involved tens of patients. Of course, any information regarding long-term effects are not going to be reliable for many years and several critical trials examining secondary risk factors are still only at their early stages.

A bit more internet-based research and suddenly that "1-in-1000" statistic quoted above (which I initially dismissed out of hand) doesn't seem so far-fetched: two deaths were reported during the clinic trials of a couple of thousand, one caused by ITP, the other by a listeria infection which led to sepsis.

The risk of ITP is now being monitored by monthly blood-tests for all lemtrada patients (which I'll need to have done for the next four years) and the risk of infection by additional advice regarding post-treatment diet and hygiene.

<u>*Thirdly, as a lemtrada patient it is important to understand the risks and the side effects that you're letting yourself in for.*</u>

To try and summarise all the NHS, and related, blurb is not easy but essentially the most important statistics would seem to be as follows:

- 2% of patients suffer, potentially very serious, autoimmune conditions with serious sounding names: immune thrombocytopenia and anti-glomerular basement membrane disease. But these risks should be mitigated by the monthly blood tests, careful monitoring and an awareness of tell-tale symptoms

- 34% suffer thyroid disorders. Initially, this figure does sound scarily high but, again, these should be identified via the monthly blood tests and can then be treated with a daily pill. Although no one would choose to have to take a daily medication for the rest of your life, this strikes me as being a bearable solution

- 71% catch post-treatment infections (17% suffer Herpes (which, I now know, is not just a STD))

- there is also a small increased risk of lymphoproliferative disorders, thyroid cancer and melanoma

In summary: 1-in-50 patients suffer extremely serious side-effects (although these should be identified early enough with careful, post-treatment blood-testing); over a third suffer serious side-effects, which then need to be managed with new drugs (which need to be taken for the rest of your life); and a majority of patients are inflicted with post-transfusion infections of some kind (to varying degrees of severity).

My ready acceptance of these risks should go to show how heavily the spectre of MS weighs upon me.

To summarise my decision:

My viewpoint is that, amongst all these statistics (*lies, damn lies and random web-based blogs*), I must remember the main pillar of my confidence: the drug has been sanctioned for use in the UK by "NICE". It has now been approved by the NHS; the FDA in the United States of America; and the EMA within Europe.

I must also remember that the option of lemtrada is a blessing, not a curse.

It is a "good" drug, here to help me.

I often think how lucky I am to have been diagnosed now rather than 10 years ago, when the only advise would have been to follow a healthy diet, yet how unlucky I am not to have been diagnosed in 10 years' time, when the current advances in stem-cell technology may have found a risk-free cure.

The NHS and the tax-payer are putting their faith in lemtrada, and in me: a daily dose of the drug costs £7,045. The full (double) treatment costs £57,000.

I hope I can look forward to many years of great health so I can start repaying some of that faith.

Pre-treatment tests: treatment minus one week

With my chemotherapy due to start in a week's time, today I had a pre-treatment appointment and was tested for any infection that might preclude the drug's use.

My progress over the last six months was discussed and reviewed. On the plus side, I have my efforts at a new diet, more focus on getting the right rest/sleep and an actual awareness of my condition. On the negative, just this last fortnight, I've been suffering a couple of most unwanted, new symptoms...

The result? Four new relapses were suggested since my initial diagnosis in March. One relapse a year signifies an MS condition that is in advance; a possible four in seven months is not great news.

It suddenly felt as though I might be losing this fight.

Left unchecked, I know that my condition will get worse and worse. Onwards it seeps – if blocked in one direction, it seems to expand in another *(an evil-spirited vapour)*. I immediately found myself mentally retreating to what I am most desperate to preserve - *the ability to walk; the ability to see* - both threatened this year. Both I do not wish to give up.

So, almost time to unleash lemtrada. A drug that eight years ago didn't exist. Fingers crossed because I feel as though I need some heavy artillery. And to toughen up. I take inspiration from those who have faced a hundred times worse with a courage that I admire.

The lemtrada decision: treatment minus one day

At times this year, I have felt as healthy as I ever have been.

I've had some wonderful times with my family, running about our new garden with my boys and out on my bike.

Cycling-wise, I've ridden in time-trials, hill races, a 600km audax and up and down some of the most famous climbs in the Alps. I've cycled 10,000 miles through hail, heavy winds, sun and rain; on ice, trails, tracks and roads; and through congested city centres and across deserted plains.

But in the seven months that have passed since my diagnosis, I have only been consistently well for perhaps eight weeks: I was happy, healthy and at my best in June; then again in September. Beyond that, most months have been patchy at best. I have had to spend far too much time being ill. There has barely been a single day since February that I haven't suffered from residual pins and needles and sensations of tingling numbness. For two, perhaps three, brief periods I've been unable to walk properly and have struggled with stairs and uneven surfaces. There were a couple of times I found myself struggling to sit up. I've briefly lost control of various muscles and of my balance and I have been scared by intermittent issues with my eyesight.

My diary reveals that I have missed 22 (twenty-two!) days of work since February through MS-related illnesses and malaise (noting that the MS-links are self-diagnosed). Career-wise, this has not been ideal but this is immaterial. It is the stresses on marital and family life that have been the most significant.

The identification of relapses is an art not a science but it feels as though I've been amassing new MS symptoms with reckless abandon. If I've had four (perhaps now five, see below) relapses in the last seven months, this needs to be compared against the average figure for annualised MS relapses, which is about 0.3. Although I don't have a calculator I can see that I've exceeded the average by some 30 times.

This last fortnight has certainly removed any doubts I might have had about my treatment. I have had another four days off work (during a critical period of my project), two new MS symptoms (that have lasted over 48 hours each so classify, by definition, as additional "MS relapses"), I'm suffering from an exhausting fatigue that has become all too familiar to me and I've been irritable at home and at work despite sleeping 11 hours a night. This latest period of "lassitude" has lasted eight days - it's nearly always 7–10 days, almost like clockwork.

In fact, for all the ups and downs of the last year, this last fortnight has been when I have felt the most "beaten". By contrast, my previous lows, bar a couple, have been offset by a surge of adrenalin, initial diagnosis included. As such, these downs have almost increased my fight, rather than reduced it, but this last relapse has just been depressing. I've been stuck in bed, frustrated. I had to miss my last cycling event of the year, which I had been tentatively training for, and my one riposte, my new MS Diet, has suddenly seemed inadequate and impotent. I've caught myself thinking, if I'm going to go down, I might as well go down stuffing myself with delicious fatty burgers and thick chocolate shakes; descending alpine passes on my bike whilst cramming my chops with creamy slices of rich carrot cake.

All-in-all this is a good time for some reinforcements to arrive, just as I appear to be flagging.

So, the lemtrada-gun gets rolled in.

I see it as a dirty, great big cannon. It's only got one bullet, this isn't a treatment you do twice.

I hope it aims carefully and with certainty.

Right between MS's eyes.

The drug's administration is not unpleasant per se (essentially, I'll be connected to an IV drip for a week), but it's not without its risks & side effects and I know that I'll have an extreme vulnerability to infection in its immediate aftermath. I approach my treatment convinced that it is the best option for me, but not without anxiety.

So, it's off to The Brain Centre, Southmead Hospital.

Time to get it done.

Let the games begin.

Battle Royale

The Fight

"Tonight.. in the corner of hope... representing the "light side" *(as well as the entire human race*)... is our newcomer and challenger.... the drug..... "**!Lemtrada!".**

Up against him – and long-time champion of the "dark side" – is the unbeaten, tour de force that is.... **"!MS!".** He will be fighting tonight, of course, with a red light-sabre that flickers with the evil flames of doom."

The Pundits

"Lemtrada is an unknown quantity. Our sources suggest he's a bit of a wild cannon *(certainly don't allow contact with your children, domestic pets... or bare skin.*)

But he certainly is a modern-day fighter: more "built" than "bred" and has spent hours and hours in the lab perfecting his one-punch style. Rumours are that he's been honed to deliver a single knock-out blow so expect him to come out hard and early. He emerged onto our NHS radar as recently as 2014 so might well have some surprises, good and bad, up his sleeve.

His explosive strength is unquestioned but does he have both the staying power and the self-control that will be needed?

Of course, we are all more familiar with MS. He has been around for over a century – and his stats speak for himself: undefeated; and apparently impregnable. The "unmoveable object". His style is certainly not for the purists – he might be attritional and steady but he is unerring.

His greatest strength is his ability to absorb attacks, nothing seems to weaken his resolve. Past opponents have been able to slow him down but he has an unparalleled ability to keep on his feet, recover and then to advance again when his opponents tire.

MS is more "ephemeral vapour" than man, so the struggle that lemtrada is going to face is how to pin him down: if you focus on one area or symptom he has a brilliant knack of exploiting another.

In lemtrada's corner is his dedicated ring-man... me.

I have prepared him as best I can through a disciplined regime of "boring, broccoli-based diet" but now, all I can do, is to supply him with the right drugs when he is suffering pain. Gabapentine, prochlorperazine, amitriptyline... boosted by steroids when required. I'll be throwing my weight behind his every punch and willing him on with my every fibre.

Lemtrada also has a strong following in the ringside seats. Row 1 sees my immediate family but there are also clusters of old friends, fellow cyclists and patients, relatives and blog-readers, many of whom are tapping away on laptops and iphones to get their up to date fight-coverage.

The followers of MS are less vocal, many of them a ghastly mist of thoughts and fears. Their support is less passionate and unquestionably more eerie but it is always there, in the corner of your eye and sub-conscience. The first few rows see "Pins and Needles" and his gaggle of team-mates: "Hypersensitivity", "Spasm" and "Numbness". This is just the family section though. Behind them, "Optic Neuritis", "Secondary Infection" and "Vertigo" are keeping a careful watch. And, in the darkened back rows of the grandstand, in apparitions hauntingly reminiscent of swirling black holes, stand the dual threats of “Immobility” and “Cognitive Loss”. The boss men. They’re drinking pints of black tar and betting wads of dirty bank notes on people’s lives as they wait to see how this fight plays itself out.”

The stakes are high.

This fight certainly has my attention.

Lemtrada Round 1: treatment done, recovery ongoing

As I left the treatment centre a week ago, I received an upbeat text: “So, you survived lemtrada!”

And so I did.

But the phrase didn’t ring quite true and this didn’t feel like a moment for a celebration. My “surviving lemtrada” feels akin to “surviving MS”, there seems to be the need to add the disclaimer, “for now.” Something slightly murky had been done to my immune system; the immediate and direct impacts of which might be fine but the endpoint is still far from known. Since then, a directly related (albeit anticipated) flare-up of my old MS symptoms has been difficult to absorb but the week of treatment, then week of recovery, has certainly given me ample time to think... maybe too much time... and so, now, I can try to piece together where I am now.

This book was always intended to intertwine MS and cycling... but I’m afraid there's ain't no cycling going on here. If I have to stretch to a cycling analogy to maintain the thread, the last fortnight has not been unlike a two week cycling adventure: there’s no way I could sum up the emotional extremes in a simple sentence; there have been some highs and lows; some tears; some pain; and, at the end of it, I’m simply back where I started.

This fortnight feels as though it’s been the confluence of many hopes and fears; big emotions that, in the immediate aftermath, I'm struggling to get on top of.

The week of my treatment

The actual facts of the treatment were perhaps the least interesting aspects of it. The drug was delivered via the steady drip of IV. Me, the patient, in bed, watching the bleeping readings of my pulse, my blood pressure and the time of day. Nurses with deep reserves of kindness asked me how I was, stuck needles in my arm and took my temperature. The drug looked no different to water but arrived each day in a black sack of thick plastic, stamped with toxicity and danger. It felt slightly cold as it went in.

The first few mornings I was given steroids first. These seemed to have the same effect as a glass of champagne, nervous before some social occasion. I don't think I'd felt so good for months, sipping a coffee, sitting up against fluffy pillows, texting friends and making bad jokes to whichever nurse happened to be within earshot. By the first afternoon though, my temperature was 38.5, my heart was pounding at 80, I was nauseous, sweaty and crawling into a ball as my head spun. But that transition on Day 1 was the worst of the week. From then on, the daily pattern became more expected and less severe. Each night I slept badly, slightly feverish, twitchy and invigorated by steroids but, each morning, I seemed to get a window of respite before the more negative side-effects arrived in the afternoon. The worst grogginess though did seem to subside each evening.

My fear that I'd get bored, stuck in a bed all week, proved unfounded but so did my hope that I'd catch up on some good books and DVDs. By the time that all my morning checks had been completed, all I felt like doing was lying, largely motionless, eyes shut but not asleep, seeing how low I could get my resting pulse.

Whilst I've never been accused of having a model's good looks, I think it's fair to say that as the week wore on I started to look quite remarkably bad... even by my own modest standards. Blotchy cold sores appeared all round my mouth and eyes and a heel-to-head, full body rash, both front and back, glowed the brightest of reds. Although these were only mild irritants, they seemed to make me all the more lethargic and tired.

It brought a wry smile to my lips when I considered quite how similar I felt to those head-crashing hangovers of my younger self: the sensation was of being slightly poisoned, drinking water to try and flush myself out. At least, this time, the drug was doing as intended, rather than some unwanted side-effect that I'd brought about through youthful craziness.

One week of treatment was certainly enough. My pallor was a tired grey and I had black rings round my eyes.

But it had been fine.

If the choice to accept this drug treatment was a decision to suffer short-term gain for long-term pain, I would have gladly suffered much worse if this would have meant an improved long-term prognosis.

As I left the hospital they ran a blood test to confirm that the lymphocyte white blood cells in my body had been completely wiped out.

The week after my treatment

I had steeled myself to feel pretty bad for a couple of weeks but not even the strongest body armour could protect me from the thoughts within.

The growing doubts – and fears.

The hardest thing to deal with hasn't been the physical side-effects but the burden of feverish ghosts and dreams. This halloween week all of my gremlins have come out to play in my fitful sleep, my fears for the future dressed up in the ridiculous white-sheets of the season. *My eyesight. My ability to walk.* I'd been warned to expect a possible relapse in my MS symptoms and so it has proved.

Several times I have had to lie down on the dining room floor as a spinning vertigo has pulled to the left... to the left... on one occasion, so violently that I bumped my head on the laminate flooring.

I trust in what I have been told - that such collective flare ups of past symptoms are not unusual - but for them to be here all together feels like a scary portent of the future. I am losing my balance when I move my eyes too swiftly from one object to another, my legs are shuddering with spasms and shakes whenever I leave them still for too long and the touch and movement of my hands seems disconnected. I have pins and needles, numbness and hypersensitivity. Lethargy. My vision feels wrong, I can't walk more than a few metres at a time and I need the loo with seconds notice.

This week, I hope, will pass (*yes – it will*) but I take it to represent what a worsened condition would be like... all the time. It feels pretty crap if this is my future... and there sure ain't no cycling going on here.

Talk and Tears

Before last week, I hadn't talked to many (or any) other MS sufferers. I hadn't really talked to many other people about my MS, full stop. Then, suddenly, all at once, there was a stream of patients sitting beside me, phone calls with old friends and family visits.

Since I was diagnosed in March, my conversations about MS have been released like my lemtrada: in little drips, a bit at a time, drops which I was happy to let go only when I had grown comfortable with their form. But this last week was like a sudden flood, inundating even my most guarded thoughts, many of which I didn't even know I had.

As other patients described their symptoms and their lives I often felt choked as they described places which maybe one day I'd go and places I'd already been. I learned that, behind whatever apparent calmness I might show, there's a pinprick of intense sensitivity that no conversation can step around: I can't be told that MS is "not so bad" and I get angry when I'm told that it is. I'm sensitive when told that "we all need to deal with it in our own way" but then I'm defensive if I'm offered advice.

There's been much introspection (too much?) this year but no tears. Then, on the Thursday, feeling swamped at a fellow patient's tale of how he slowly had to give up his job and then his mobility, for the first time I felt my eyes prickle. At that moment another visitor, I suppose trying to help, interjected with how terrible a condition MS was.

"A friend of mine has terminal cancer. They say they'd much rather have the certainty of cancer than suffer a deteriorating MS for the rest of their lives."

The exchange had made me wobbly with a disproportionate irritation. I called an old friend of mine who lives many miles away and he listened to me talk for more time on a phone than I probably have done for many years combined. Emotions tugged away. My bed began to feel like some lifeless capsule cut adrift from my actual life, some non-descript corner of some foreign field, far from home.

The nurses, suddenly and obviously, were not my family and I felt as though I was being experimented on by white jackets.

I badly wanted to see my wife. And my boys.

When the nurse next attended, I seemed to have shed a few silent tears. By the way, I found rumours that tears are cathartic to be unfounded. They left me with a headache and a sore throat.

"Don't worry... it's the steroids," she said. "They give you the baby blues."

"What's the cure to those?"

"The only known one is no baby in the first place..."

All this talking was proving too emotional for me. The last thing I needed was to get started thinking about my boys...

Now I just want this window of treatment/recovery to end – I've had enough of it – and I want to get back on with my life.

Three weeks post-lemtrada: Teaching an old dog new tricks

Three weeks since lemtrada and I'm still largely housebound. I'm deeply frustrated by my current lethargies and am not dealing too brilliantly with this relative immobility.

When asked how I am, I complain about an ongoing issue with my eyesight, a debilitating vertigo that seems to strike three or four times day, almost dragging me to the floor, and I mention an ongoing exhaustion, which I can't seem to shake. But what I'm struggling to cope with the most is inside my head. Inside I'm so angry at these lost days, these opportunities at life which are passing me by.

I can't help but wonder whether it's the same for everyone or whether, for some reason, I'm particularly ill-suited to these changes or just stubbornly unable to accept them.

My two boys wrestle on the floor. Again.

They're incessant bundles of frenetic energy and don't seem to do much else.

There's a four year gap between them, a space that the younger one furiously tries to bridge on determined repeat.

Although they've been brought up the same way, they are undeniably different boys *(special, of course, in their own ways!).* Who knows which brief moments in time have most formed their personalities and which strands of their DNA pushed them one way rather than another? Whatever "they are", of course, they come, at least, in part, from me.

From a young age I, too, have always had a restlessness. What is becoming all too clear is that, however I was born – whatever it is that I am now – I'm certainly not well-equipped for being a patient. I feel that there is some poorly understood process within me, something that compels me to get up at 4am on a rainy February morning to cycle 200km, that sits particularly poorly with being largely housebound for, what is now, 22 consecutive days.

In fact, it's driving me mad.

What gives me the compulsion to get up at 4am and cycle 200km? It's a worry that I might miss out. I hate the feeling of life passing me by and, at the moment, it feels as though it's slipping through my fingers at the rate of knots.

Reading more about MS, and the possible behavioural traits associated with it, a "nervous energy" is described as being particularly typical. I don't like the term "nervous energy", it feels negative and implies some sort of anxiety, unease or dissatisfaction, none of which I want to relate to. Maybe I'm extrapolating my own paranoid sensitivities but it also seems to imply a certain degree of self-centredness, whirring on my own hamster-wheel at a different pace to others, and I don't like that thought.

But, although I might not like it, in parts, I confess, the cap does seem to fit.

And, as I get older, I do wonder if it's getting worse.

After I left school, my back-packing days, which were seminal times for me, certainly didn't bring me to a calmer acceptance of my place in world. Instead, the most significant perspective I seemed to glean was of the temporal fragility of it all and how I was to be forever fated to miss so much more than I could ever see. This panic of mortality only enhanced my desire to see and do as much as possible, as quickly as possible, before it all turned to dust.

It feels as though I now need to learn some new techniques for life because the philosophies and life-skills that I have slowly developed don't seem to be so appropriate anymore. Maybe I have to consciously unravel a bit of what I am and teach myself to change.

I don't want valium to the be the answer to it all.

Four weeks post-lemtrada: On a bike, not at work

Lemtrada plus four weeks.

I am improving. I am getting there but it feels like progress is very slow.

Last weekend, for the first time, I was out on a bike. It felt a bit wobbly (I felt a bit wobbly) but it was hugely uplifting to feel some fresh air on my face. Things were definitely moving in the right direction. Turning glass-pedals, wrapped in layer upon layer to keep out the cold, I, at last, felt as though things were going to be OK.

The air was crystal clear and the sky was blue.

Happiness seemed so uncomplicated.

To add a sense of challenge to my lemtrada treatment, the last few weeks have seen, firstly, a house move; and then, secondly, my wife losing her job. As is often the case, timing could probably have been better. This undercurrent (over-current?) of stress has been somewhat exacerbated by the fact that I'm not getting any sick-pay during this current period of recovery. I've long benefitted from the freedoms of being self-employed but sadly sick-pay is not one of them. With all this in mind, I made a bid today to get back to work. The financial imperative.

It did not go well.

In fact, it started to go wrong before I'd even arrived at the office. As I tentatively commuted in by car, another driver crashed into me whilst I sat stationary at some lights. A crumpled bonnet, smashed number plate and a sore neck & head. It could have been worse, I'm lucky I wasn't on my bike.

When I did belatedly actually get to work, I couldn't remember my laptop's six-digit user ID - the same ID I'd used every day at work for over a year. I then worried that my brain had been turned irreparably to mush... then further panicked when I couldn't remember my colleague's name... I wondered how long I could hope to maintain the pretence of a job if my mind had actually ceased to function...

Despite leaving home a good hour early, I was then running late and had to hurry to my appointed training session without having lunch. I was due to run a training session of perhaps 15 attendees.

I didn't have any time to prepare and was talking to my audience before I'd really had a chance to compose myself. It quickly became apparent that I couldn't focus on my screen. I was trying to use my laptop as I illustrated points on an OHP but the focus, then re-focus, on more than one screen was too much for me and the dreaded vertigo kicked in. I started to hear, and then listen to, my own voice as though it was somehow disconnected from anything I was doing. A thought flashed into my head that maybe I was dreaming... and then a second later a panic that I was maybe going to faint. Mid-sentence, I paused... sat down... then announced that I couldn't continue. A colleague gamely stepped in as I exited stage-right and adopted the brace position.

I wondered if I could get away with charging two minutes of time for the period that I had actually been talking. I wondered if I'd be able to get back home safely. I felt very ill.

Happiness can be so uncomplicated. What a shame that we can't always just be so.

Six weeks post-lemtrada: The Force Awakens. A New Hope

I have not found it easy, these last six weeks, post-lemtrada.

I've been struggling with vertigo, a deep-seated fatigue and general malaise.

I very much acknowledge that, in some ways, I was probably not making things easy for myself. I couldn't come to peace with my new predicament. I burned with frustrations and cabin fever and I couldn't resist over-doing things when I did feel OK. Although I acknowledged these flaws, I failed to compensate for them and couldn't seem to alter my emotions or behaviours. The fact that I couldn't even change those things within my power makes me feel a bit embarrassed and full of fuss.

My head knew that I was still alive and well, happy with my two healthy children. My spirit, though, felt angry and battling, reeling in a fight.

Then, on Monday this week, I got out of bed and for the first time in over a month, I didn't immediately have to pause for my legs and arms to stop shaking with spasms. I walked to the bathroom and, for the first time in over a month, I didn't immediately feel awash with vertigo. I commuted into Bristol and, just about, did half a day's work (although even this was cut-short at lunchtime by pretty overwhelming bout of dizziness).

On Tuesday, I took my winter bike around some of the local canal paths. My vision was disorientating and I felt dizzy and tired but this definitely counted as a bike ride, in the rain. I had so missed fresh air.

On Thursday, I cycled up a hill for the first time in many weeks. I might have felt as weak as a kitten but this was how things would get re-started.

Fast-forward to today, Saturday, and I've now got a full day's work under my belt and I'm contemplating the start-line (maybe the ride?) for tomorrow's charity bike ride with my club, Bristol South.

I've had a few more glitches. I had the embarrassment of completely losing my balance as I stepped out of a lift at work and vertigo continues to kick-in from time to time during innocent conversations. I'm certainly not "back", not yet, but it now feels as though I'm on the right road. It was when I was able to get out on a bike again that my mood changed. My spirit improved almost immediately and I could feel my internal engine kicking into gear once more. I feel as though my will, my hopes and my optimism have returned. In the absence of being able to walk, let alone jog or run, this is why cycling has become so important to me.

My life-force.

Last night I booked us family tickets for the new Star Wars film.

"The Force Awakens" indeed.

Game on, 2016. Full of "A New Hope".

Three months post-lemtrada: The body feels ahead of the mind

Three months post-lemtrada. Maybe this is just another man-made line in the sand but it has added significance because I'd been steeling myself for what I'd been told might be up to 90 days of physical depletion after my treatment.

It was mid-February last year when I had last walked painlessly and freely. At my worst, I could barely walk at all. At my best, there was still a mechanical clunkiness that I struggled to articulate. I had an awareness that something felt a bit wrong, stiff, wobbling and robotic, and I had an ever-present undercurrent of pins and needles.

Then, last Sunday, as my boys ran pretty aimlessly around a rugby field, it dawned on me that some sort of spring had returned to my step. I equate the sensation with the looseness brought on by a particularly successful physio-visit or yoga session. I don't know when exactly it happened but, suddenly, I was having to consciously search to find the smallest hint of pins and needles. I found that I was "striding" again rather than "shuffling", as I'd become so used to.

And I've been back on my bike. I've been back, riding with friends, who I can, just about, keep up with, thinking how much fun all this is and how much I'd miss it if it went away. The body is creaking as I remind it what cycling is about. I have aches here and there, my old arthritic knee, troublesome sciatica and no "kick" in my legs, but these are all obstacles I understand and have been long frustrated by. Although there's no short-cut around them, they do not carry with them the more sinister, hidden, threat of MS.

Getting back into my cycling isn't proving that easy. Nor, perhaps, do I want it be. I've "bonked" a few times already (the term cyclist's use to describe that unwanted sensation when suddenly the body can cycle no more – an absolute crash in energy levels that is insurmountable) and have returned from a couple of shorter rides disconcertingly late due to my average speed. Even my commute home is taking noticeably longer than I remember. But I do want to get back that feeling of being capable and free. I don't want to get used to a new, reduced norm.

In the book, "Life of Pi", Pi describes his family's experiences of owning an Indian zoo in the seventies. On the rare occasion that an animal would escape its captivity, the most common result was not that the animal would run amok, nor make a bee-line for the freedoms of the wilderness, instead, after a few tentative circles of new territory, it would typically return to its cage, where it felt safe, in familiar surrounds, and would await its next meal.

My latest worry is about the fogginess of mind that I've been experiencing the last few weeks. I gather that this is not unfamiliar post-lemtrada, so I keep my fingers crossed that it will pass. At the moment, I can still see the funny side: discussing deadlines with a colleague, I spent at least five minutes thinking (mid-January) that we were already in March; I enjoyed a dinner party with my wife, but realised afterwards that I couldn't remember a single person's name round the table; and I have been forgetting not only names of prominent celebrities and actors, but of old friends too, let alone the names of their children or partners. Maybe this is all just me growing old... maybe not. I do see on the internet that many people in my position have similar concerns, but, coupled with the occasional bout of disabling vertigo, I wonder how much longer I can retain the mask of competent employee...

Always remember not to let MS be your excuse for everything. It is no less "you" than the scar on your cheek, colour of your hair or love for your children.

Brain Fog

The season is slowly hinting at the very first signs of spring, but my own small shoots of recovery seem to have been a bit of a false dawn. After a couple of weeks of tentative cycling, I've been bedbound again.

I've been off-work. I've felt empty and sapped – dizzy and tired with those now familiar, incessant rumblings of vertigo and blurry vision.

Another 10 days off my bike.

These symptoms of malaise aren't easy to articulate. "I'm not feeling great," is the lament my wife keeps hearing. I'm struggling for the right words and my brain feels tired.

It feels like there's a glitch in the matrix or wrinkle in space-time. It is clicking like a badly indexed rear derailleur, searching for the right gear to run smooth again.

Like the emperor's new clothes, everyone else seems to be continuing as normal, so I question whether it is only me that senses we are all in a dream....

Like when the soundtrack to a film falls slightly out of line with the scene at play and it takes a while to work out quite what's wrong...

Like I'm dreaming a series of deja-vus.

I feel like there's a dark spot in me, which is ironic because the MRI scans highlight them as spots of brilliant white – like they are cleansing drips of something pure, rather than dotted warnings of decay.

As the dust from another house move this year settles, I unpack another box of old photos.

Pictures of me as a child: pointing at ice cream in the garden or wrapped up in gloves in the snow.

I show my own children. That was me. The very same me, many dreams ago. I remember a memory of seeing those photos before... and I remember remembering how they were once taken.

I show them photos of me backpacking around the world. I remember those places too but I look so young. My skin seems translucent compared to now. Although I could never see it at the time, it's now clear to me just how much my eyes look the same as my cousins'.

I remember being hungry as I tightened my budget. I remember eating pancakes on the beach.

But I was a different person then. It seems like a world away.

London in my twenties now blurs with my days at school. One of my flatmates from that time was also one of my best friends from my teens. He visited me here, at home, a fortnight ago, which somehow added to this feeling of other-worldliness. I couldn't catch whether his face had changed from when he was 13 or 27. I hugely enjoyed his company but we weren't the same people as we were a decade ago. There are photos of us on night's out that I don't remember being taken.

There's also a photo of me taken minutes before my son was born. I don't remember that being taken either – but, again, what strikes me is how young my eyes are... how young my face was. I catch myself thinking, hasn't that just happened? But it was almost 10 years ago – those days of living in Cardiff now feel like a dream.

We lived in Australia. I remember the smell of my favourite coffee shop and the sign on its door, but not what it looked like inside.

I remember cooking lemon cheesecake with my son but the fact that he was only two years old feels like a disconnect. In photos I look tanned, and I don't have a beard. I muse that I would never have known then where I would be living now.

Living in Bristol was only two years ago but it seems no more recent than my days in London. I check again, puzzled that these memories are not fresher as they are more recent but they all feel like a bit of a haze. I remember feeling very, very tired and lying down on the kitchen floor... or maybe I just remember a photo I've seen of me doing that, my boys laughing that I should get up.

We have lived in our current place for two years too, but I can't picture in my mind's eye what it was like when we arrived... or what we were like. I do some mental arithmetic which confirms that we had our two boys then but these memories could easily sit a decade ago... before, or after, London... or Cardiff... or Australia.

Only last week, I was cycling to work but even this memory seems no more recent than those times I used to ride along a beach outside Fremantle, Western Australia. I had a moment when I almost 'came to' as I pedalled, like I'd just woken up. Momentarily I couldn't remember where I was going and, at that point in time, I could have been on that Western Australian cycle path... or riding across Battersea Park... or in bed, asleep, having this dream. I stared at the road in front of me and the sensation passed after maybe 10-15 seconds... it was a Wednesday in Bristol. I checked my back-pocket and, yes, my Staff ID pass was still there. The early morning darkness was of late-February, not October nor November.

I feel that something isn't quite right.

Like I'm living a series of deja-vus.

The school run today was fairly standard. I battled with my younger son for ten minutes to get him to wear his jumper and we eventually kerfuffled out of the house a few minutes late. Upon arrival at the school gates, he was just in his T-shirt again.

I walked back home, got the jumper and went back to school again.

Nothing had really moved on. The same parents were there. I couldn't remember whether I'd already said hello to them... or thought that I was about to, or just had... or was I just remembering the sight of them from five minutes earlier?

I think I'm tired. And need to sleep. Trying to think is making me more so – like the thoughts that I'm trying to catch keep accelerating, tantalisingly just beyond my reach. I forget whatever it was I was trying to think of so return instead to a mental list of tick-boxes in order to satisfy myself with where I am and when.

I lost my mobile phone which I left, I think, at a playground in Corsham as I pushed my boys on a swing.

Those photo albums don't seem to make much sense, let alone matter anymore.

The past of bright eyes and youthful face.

The trees outside this window have started to show little buds of green, just this last couple of days.

The seasons are turning.

Déjà-vu.

I remember spending a week of summer holiday up in Scotland with my Granny.

"Weeks go by so quickly, Granny," I said.

"At my age," she replied, "it's the decades that disappear."

I google quotes from Buddhism: "do not dwell in the past, do not dream of the future. Concentrate the mind on the present moment," and, after 10 days off, I get on my bike again. I felt very ill.

Inception

Saito: *Have you come to kill me? I've been waiting for someone...*

Cobb: *Someone from a half-remembered dream.*

Saito: *Cobb? Impossible. We were young men together. I'm an old man.*

Cobb: *Filled with regret...*

Saito: *Waiting to die alone...*

Cobb: *I've come back for you... to remind you of something. Something you once knew...*

Cobb: *That this world is not real. To take a leap of faith. Come back... so we can be young men together again. Come back with me...*

I'm young still. These murmurings of discontent must pass.

Four months post-lemtrada: Keep going

Four months post-lemtrada.

No spells of vertigo for over a week.

And, today, a bike ride that was as good as it gets. Clear, windless, blue skies, cold, fresh air and me feeling strong, fit and happy to be alive. Those weeks and weeks of grimacing through stormy winds and tough winter rain, weakness and dizziness, all now feel worthwhile. The bike felt fast and light, I felt free and high on adrenalin.

This is why I want to cycle through MS. And, touch wood, long may I do so.

This feels like the date that the chemo-drugs have, at last, been flushed from my system. Free in the fresh air again I had to wipe away tears.

Game on, the rest of my life.

All MS patients are different, and have their own variants of the condition, but my experience of MS-illness runs a pretty consistent pattern. Often, if not always, I go through a period when I feel as though there is no end in sight and that the relapse has become my new "normal". I cease to remember not being tired and have tears in my eyes for no reason at random times of day. I burn with cabin fever and frustration and itch at life passing me by.

I now write of my pleasure at this short bike ride, not so much for others to read but for myself, to re-read in the future the next time I feel down, to, hopefully, take optimism and strength from it.

So, to my future me, things will be fine. Toughen up, pal, you can beat this.

Keep going.

Five months later, Day 38 of a latest malaise, I re-read the above, desperate to start believing again when I most need to.

I read the words but I don't seem to have any energy to harness their power.

Right now, I feel like a blue badge holder... and definitely not a professional, father, husband or friend. Let alone an alpine cyclist, laughing with friends as we race up little climbs and breathe in the fresh air of new views. These joys feel so removed and long-distant from where I now am. I have to learn some better techniques of keeping faith because these repeated bouts of malaise continue to get me down, too much so to be sustainable.

Keep going.

Bruno

When I was just a boy I had to spend some time in Whittington Hospital just before Christmas. To the excitement of the children's ward, Frank Bruno arrived in full Santa's attire to distribute presents and send our spirits soaring. A free-standing, inflatable Bruno punch-bag was put up for the great man to demonstrate his punching power and for the children to then emulate. The huge smiling face of Bruno himself adorned the target as child after child took a hit at him and watched him enthusiastically bounce back up – again and again. Again and again he'd be hit but his smile refused to fade. This huge, great big, teethy grin would pop back up for the next child to knock back down.

Pop / bounce / grin / pop / bounce / grin.

I wonder where behind that smile were the tears and pain that we couldn't see.

Pop. Then up again. Still smiling.

I look you in the eyes, MS. Still smiling, ready – if need be – to be hit again.

Keep going.

I try not to consider the fact that my second dose of lemtrada is now only eight months away.

Chapter Seven: Chemo-cycling

Building blocks and curve balls

My lemtrada treatment was to be split into two sets of infusions, one year apart: October to October. Come that first mid-December, I was beginning to daydream about what I might be able to do that summer. My immune system continued to go about its job, frantically replenishing my lymphocyte cells into a semblance of working order. I could only hope that it knew what it was doing.

I've always quite liked the clean-slate feeling of a new calendar.

It represents possibilities and potential: there's all that empty room for plans and dreams that haven't yet been squeezed out by the passage of time.

When I was a young backpacker I remember getting the same buzz of excitement as I stood, starry-eyed, in Paris's Gare du Nord. Rather than the humdrum names of Slough, Daventry, Swindon or Barnstaple, the Departure Board was crammed full of new adventures: Barcelona and Brussels; St Petersburg or Bucharest; Budapest and Vienna.

It was as if all boundaries had been removed.

I know that there are textbooks that'll tell you that January 1st is but "a Western construct" and represents nothing more than an arbitrary line in the sand (*why wasn't the line drawn at midnight on the shortest day to tally with the spinning of the planets and stars?*) but I quite like it the way it is. What couldn't be done last year, becomes possible again. Things can be rectified or restarted.

Over Christmas, my recovery from lemtrada treatment was moving in the right direction. Bouts of vertigo ceased being daily. Some force deep inside me, my internal engine, began to give off little sparks again, trying to catch alight. I slept nine hours a night and slowly turned pedals on my bike. There were a couple of unwanted moments when my balance disappeared – in a waiting room, in a restaurant and on a plane – but these were the exceptions, rather than the rule.

Since New Year, I've found myself glancing at lists of cycling events, like exotic destinations on that departure board: the Alps and Snowdonia; audaxes and day-tours.

At the moment though, these have to remain as mere sparks. They are always immediately followed by a reflection of my ongoing physical weaknesses and tiredness of fight.

Of course, it is the element of surprise that makes a curve ball such a good weapon:

Last Sunday, I donned my winter jacket, waterproof gloves, winter leggings and snood and headed out for my first long(ish) ride since my treatment.

I wondered what my body held in store for me.

A couple of hours later, as I rode on the A36, an on-coming motorist, who cannot have seen me, accelerated furiously into my lane as he overtook at what I'd guess to be 50mph+ in wet conditions.

There was simply no room on the road for both me and him and I was forced into the tall roadside kerb, which I momentarily scraped along before toppling over.

I wasn't hurt, apart from a slightly sprained wrist and the indignity of a scratch of dirt up my left-hand side, but I'd suffered not only a front wheel blow-out, but also a two inch slit in the tyre itself.

I tried, as best I could, to use the ripped inner tube to fashion an emergency tyre patch that would get me to the nearest bike shop early on a Sunday morning.

Ultimately, I got a new tyre, got back on my bike and finished my ride... just. No endurance. No stamina.

Not yet.

But my struggle was not with MS, it was with poor conditioning and an absence of training.

Hard work. But if it wasn't? Well.... everybody would be doing it wouldn't they?

My first building block of 2016, albeit a slightly wobbly one.

Footnote: *It's almost exactly a year since the last time I was hit, head-on, by a motorist as she drove up the wrong side of the road in Bristol. I still await any compensation for my injuries and all the damage that was done. Pleading guilty in the subsequent court case, the driver was fined £120 and given a suspended ban from driving.*

Further footnote*: Last year, a speed camera captured me, very early in the morning, driving my car at 37mph along a deserted, straight and dry Welsh road, designated as a 30, For this, I, too, was fined £120 and had 3 penalty points added to my licence.*

The "Brevet Cymru" 400km audax (again)

Last weekend, I cycled the Brevet Cymru 400km, again. But this time, post-chemotherapy.

What hadn't changed was that it was still a long time to be riding a bike.

So much road rolled under my wheels that early preoccupations at the start of the ride later reappeared as dream-like deja-vues. In the very depths of the night, the line between consciousness and sleep seemed to blur as I wondered whether my thoughts were merely echoing whispers I'd already heard before.

Riding largely solo, I began to fear that the sights and sounds were coming too thick and fast for me to accurately describe later, the whole experience began to seem like an anchorless and discombobulated drift of time. I could scarcely believe that it had started only 24 hours earlier. Like always on a ride of that length, my thoughts crept into new realisations and perspectives; and questions of why I was doing what I was doing - under the night skies - and for whom.

Distinct memories now seem like little pin-pricks in an otherwise swelling, ebbing and flowing mass of non-discernible progress through field and glen, valley and climb:

A red kite hovered above me, several more observed my passing-by; and a large heron glided alongside without so much of a twitch of its wings. A collie ran alongside the small group I had joined, playfully pacing our peloton for mile after mile, waiting for us when he had sprinted too far ahead.

A massive tractor slammed on its horn as I wheeled around a tight right-angled bend straight into its bull-dozing path.

Other riders overtook me with little quips of conversation and, from time-to-time, I sat with other cyclists as their speed fell into step with mine.

I stopped for coffees, energy drinks, bananas and beans, breaks which punctuated all those roads-upon-roads in between. At these break-stops, I sometimes saw myself through others' eyes: small groups of friends looking at this solo rider wondering if they should risk inviting him in to their well-balanced units of pedal and chat. I didn't know whether I should brazenly tag-along or keep an introverted distance.

And, of course, I have MS.

I thought very much about my wife and my children and about how, until a few days earlier, I had still been struggling to break-out of the malaise from my latest MS relapse. I thought about how staying up too late was making me anxious as to the repercussions the next day and about how little imbalances of temperature, tiredness or stress would exacerbate the buzz of pins and needles in my hands and feet.

I had just come out of the back of it and here I was, looking at the sea on the West Wales Coast, about to start cycling another 100 miles, through the night, to get back home.

I felt healthy but the folly of this was there for all to see. I had no (or virtually no) MS symptoms but, as the sun set and the temperature suddenly dropped, the event felt more and more like something irresponsible for me to be doing. Soon after I left the coast,, of course, I found myself lost. With that feeling of dawning realisation all seasoned cyclists must recognise, I went through that familiar, but painful, process: having to admit to myself that I didn't know where I was; quell the disappointment;

and then get on with putting it right. I accidently added 17km to the route on that leg and it chipped away at my resolve.

The night, however, was a pretty perfect one. A huge long descent on the beautifully smooth A40 was helped by a light tailwind. The temperature dropped to near-freezing and, as a result, the air was crisply clear and the stars were all out to shine. It was in these early hours of the morning though that the ride became its hardest. This was probably just a well-trained body-clock beginning to cry for sleep but one of the side-effects of such a long descent were that the chills had really set in. My energy levels dropped through the floor and things started to swim and swirl. I was grateful when a much cheerier rider pulled me in and allowed me to rather doggedly draft him home, tiptoeing past some wheel-spinning joy-riders fresh from a night out in Abergavenny town.

I had ridden the whole audax with the one-legged lop-sidedness that I have now adopted. New cycling shoes, new foot-beds, heavy strapping and anti-inflammatories all internet-researched weapons against the issues I'd been having with my left foot. My joints were swollen but not unduly. My concern was that my left foot was still curled up in its curiously apologetic way when I got home.

Conclusions

As the last few miles went by, I reflected on how lucky I felt. How lucky – and how deeply happy – I was to be alive. To have MS and to be out on my bike... how grateful I was. I acknowledged more than ever before that I couldn't risk blowing such a good hand. I will continue riding my bike but these crazy rides through the night are not worth the risk anymore. Pins and needles were back in my hands and left arm and these through-the-nighters cannot be considered to be worth it given my other loves and responsibilities.

I also reflected how, again, I'd been nuzzled along by the kindness of strangers: the (nameless?!) cyclist who shepherded me home, chatting to keep me awake whilst he dropped his own speed to meet mine; and a fellow called Ben who patiently helped me tease a shard of glass out of my tyre having found me rather covered in oil, failing to get the job done myself.

"Net Net" I had to confess, in my audaxing days I'd certainly been helped more by strangers than I had helped them and I figure that the same could probably also be said of my life. If my final conclusion is that I should always give more than I take that's perhaps an honourable point to come to an end. If I can live up to it of course.

Chemo-seasons

I've been reading my son the "Little House on the Prairie" series. As our own house buzzes with umpteen electronic devices – from can openers to Ipads to espresso machines to toothbrushes – the books feel like bygone writings about bygone eras. Set in the deep mid-West of the USA, the Wilder family battle against the elements to try and to eke out a simple, subsistence lifestyle that survives winter blizzards, summer droughts, prairie fires and locust swarms.

Living in the modern-day UK, I would say that the seasons rotate around our lives, not vice versa. On my bike, I like this revolution and enjoy the act of cycling through all the weathers. Their passing punctuates chapters of time and of life, day by day, month by month, I envisage our planet spinning in its elliptical orbit in freefall round the sun.

On my first ride of 2016, the roads felt bald, polished by night-time frosts. I couldn't trust their gleaming surfaces; winks of black ice amongst the pretty coating of white dust. The morning darkness felt as though it might crack with cold. The Milky Way could be seen, crisp and clear in the sky, an innocent, silent witness to our lives, light years below. Despite double-gloves and shoe covers, my fingers and toes smarted with a swollen numbness and my body raged with the prickles of MS when I had a hot showers.

Six months later, I rode my bike through the Alps. I rested, exhausted and panting on my handlebars as a stream of sweat poured down from my face. My eyes stung with salt; my lightweight summer cycling-top was soaking wet. I was drinking my water more quickly than I could get to the next water-stop and my arms and legs were pasted with layers of suncream and dust. I had started to get cramps in my inner thigh and the soles of my feet were burning hot pressure points. The dominant smell was that of tarmac which felt soft and sticky as it melted under a blazing sun. I had just passed by a digital temperature display showing 39.4 degrees. There wasn't a breath of wind. The Alps felt raw. Beautiful. Uncompromising[4]. And hot.

In between these two rides, as seems to be a recurring annual pattern, my MS had flared up, dragging me down; it had then stutteringly abated, before, with a realisation similar to that of watching the tidal retreat on my bike in Pwll last week, it suddenly dawned on me that I couldn't see the waves anymore. The surf that had been lapping at my toes just a moment ago was now only rock pools. A few eddying currents remained but the estuary shimmered with the ripples of sand, not water. A convoy of beach vehicles drove where, an hour earlier, the sea had stood. Somehow I hadn't even noticed it retreating.

This year, my toughest day of cycling in the Alps saw me ascend almost 6,500 metres. I drank ten litres of water but still finished the ride feeling dehydrated and sun-struck. When my alarm rang at 6am the following morning, I felt drained and empty but I was not buzzing with pins and needles. Tiredness and pins & needles I had grown to see almost as being one and the same but not this time. I mentally turned the physical pages of my own body: a

---

[4] *I'm slightly embarrassed to have used this word. My experience of the Alps was only as "uncompromising" as a tourist-trap with hot coffees and fresh pastries can be!*

residual tingling in toes and fingers and in my left abdomen and an urgent, and familiar, need to suddenly go to the toilet... but nothing worse.

Perhaps a 200km Alpine bike ride is in fact the cure afterall.

Continuing that bike tour when physically empty allowed for only steady, slow progress, whilst trying to allow the body to regenerate on the bike. Eating, drinking, resting... avoiding the midday sun. I did feel stronger the next day but the remaining three days were all on go-slow. Go-slow may be, but no MS.

That tour felt like the making hay of summer. Like Mr Wilder in those books, this was me, reaping the harvest of a winter's hard-work.

Weirdly, and perhaps paradoxically, a few days later I managed to flare-up my MS by jogging no more than ten metres alongside my boys. Pins and needles were back up my torso and arms; a grey pallor to my face, a strange disconnectedness to my left-foot and a few days of buzzy exhaustion followed. One time, I had to lie down with vertigo after simply looking upwards into some trees. This was a reminder that I have to watch it carefully, this hiding friend of mine - but I do believe that summertime is "my time". It always has been.

The months pass. The seasons rise and fall. My MS ebbs and flows. I wonder where my new "normal" now sits. Like our earth spinning in the universe, I must remember that my MS is just a small part of a wider whole and so very much more is going on. Make hay while I can, let's see what next winter brings.

Hindsight

Any gambler knows the sensation. *"if only I'd just bet on 19..." "I was going to..." "I normally always..."*

I have it with my Fantasy League Football Team... *"I was going to put in Aguero..." "I was just about to make Rooney my captain"...*

And there's that urban legend of the lottery player whose direct debit ran out and no ticket was bought, the week before their regular numbers came up on a Saturday night.

I have just finished listening to Series Two of the radio-podcast, "Serial" *(highly recommended)* which had a whole episode called "Hindsight" and spent most of its 11 hours chewing over the unintended consequences and ramifications of a single action. Lives can change, of course, based on just one phone-call. One word said and not rescinded. One drink too many. One hug too few.

Of course, all our lives are made up of if not infinite, certainly countless, decisions or choices. The huge majority are never given even a second thought – which spoon to take from the cutlery drawer; which pair of socks to put on – others demand more contemplation: our builders are (still!) building an attic extension in our new house; I've just started a new contract working in Bristol; and my second bout of chemotherapy is booked in for seven weeks' time.

The continuous flow of the smaller decisions does sometimes catch a snag and becomes memorable as a result – *if only I had turned left not right; answered that phone-call; or left the house a minute later* - but you can't dally on their process, these choices need to be made continuously and quickly, almost sub-consciously as a by-product of "what we do". *No less so than the beating of our hearts.*

It is our bigger, conscious decisions that are more likely to be followed by reflection. Hopefully a happy one, but sometimes rueful, sometimes with regret. If bigger decisions, whatever their details, can be a framed with your own "worldview" or "moral compass" at least as regrets will be of chance outcome, fate or bad luck, rather than process.

Bear with me here because the line that divides the uncritical acceptance of one, versus the conscious review of the other is an interesting one. At one time in my life, my nine-to-five job had become a daily flow but, when I recognised it as an active "decision", I changed instead to self-employment, where I've been ever since. In theory, most of life could probably be deconstructed in this way, revisiting the sub-conscious to make them conscious: the house you live in; the town.... even the country... or hemisphere; your marriage or your friends. Of course, you'd feel paralysed if you critiqued all these big decisions all the time so they have to become the backdrop to your day-to-day.

Yesterday I chatted to a friend who has just had a baby and is moving homes. And jobs. And so is his wife. And they've recently moved countries. He would confirm that his current status quo is probably unsustainable.

It has struck me this last week that a couple of my recent, really big decisions had got a bit lost in my own "flow". I had forgotten that they were choices at all:

This year, I've insisted on continuing to cycle.

I've cycled because I enjoy it. Love it, in fact.

Because I've been struggling to walk.

Because, at times, my head has felt so clogged with stresses, emotions and confusion that I've needed to.

Because it's what I do.

I've cycled to work. And have "gone for a cycle" on a weekend. *Left foot; right foot; pedal pedal pedal; click click, gear change; pedal pedal.*

Cycling has become a barometer for my MS. At times, I've been numb with buzzing pins and needles and weakness whilst, at others, I've felt so fit and on top of the world that I could laugh out loud. I've had tears in my eyes at both extremes. I've been scared of losing it and desperately keen to make the most of it whilst I still can.

This week, I cycled my 10,000th mile of the year. Boosted by spring-time audaxing and summer-time touring, that averages out at over 40miles a day, riding in wind, rain, sleet and hail, as well as in glorious sunshine. Up and down, vale and hill.

I didn't set out to reach this figure. I set out to ride where I could, when I could, scared by the looming black cloud of MS. A cloud which could, at some random God-given point, bring it all to a close.

This weekend, though, I did not ride my bike.

10,000 miles felt like enough.

I wonder if cycling is indeed just "what I do". Or whether I should revisit my choice to do it so much.

"Hindsight"

I think back to 18 months or so ago.

I realise now how much adrenalin (or stress) I was cycling with. My MS diagnosis was new and I was cycling with fight. Living with fight and perhaps with a barely simmering frustration.

I saw cycling as my offence (and defence) and my means of a comeback.

But, as they all said it would, the confusion and fear of those initial months did fade. My condition is now "my MS", rather than a new diagnosis. I better know what elements of it can be fought and beaten *(or maybe I just think I do?)*; and I'm still seeking to come to terms with those bits which cannot.

I do feel as though I've cycled away several knots in my mind and now have fewer fears that I need to make peace with. Mulling them over and over whilst out on the bike has helped to smooth away many jagged edges and jarring cuts.

10,000 miles.

At times, my legs turned the pedals – *left foot, right foot* – as subconscious a flow as the beating of my heart. It was a meditation as I felt blood move through my veins and my lungs empty, then fill with air.

Perhaps it's what I do because it's what I have to.

And my current hindsight? The one, indirectly ms-related decision I wish I could go back and change? Like that gambler who bets on red not black, I rue never having invested in any professional illness cover or insurance. I rue all those days this year when I've been unable to earn an income. As the main income-earner in my family, I worry about what the future may hold. Insurance is always worth it with hindsight after the event.

There is no "fair"

The event that precipitated my MS diagnosis was caused by a motorist accelerating up the wrong side of a road in Central Bristol. They hit me head-on as I was commuting to work on my bike.

My bike was hit so hard that only its rear cassette, crank-arms and pedals would be salvageable.

My only items of clothing that were not written-off were my socks - even these had their blood stains - and my right shoe.

By all accounts, the driver was shocked and apologetic.

The police did their enquiries, solicitors got involved and the chain of paperwork started.

The costs of replacing the bike were relatively easy to quantify but how to put a value on all the other injuries, stresses, flashbacks and scarring? Let alone the extent to which my MS was exacerbated with implications for both my short-term health and long-term prognosis.

At last, it now seems that a settlement has been agreed but it is difficult to say whether the amount is “fair”. When you add up my direct losses and equipment damage etc *(which I priced very conservatively using discount websites)* the value of compensation for my injuries and stress can be deduced as being around £5,000. I now somewhat regret pricing my equipment losses so modestly given that many of the replacements I ended up buying were more expensive than what I had claimed. Apparently, a cheque will be arriving within a couple of months.

Last week, a friend of mine was hit as a car pulled out directly in front of her in Bristol, a classic SMIDSY ("Sorry, mate, I didn't see you"). A broken helmet and an ambulance call-out.

Less than two months ago, another friend was knocked-off in very similar circumstances and is currently still recovering from her broken collar bone.

On Friday morning, as I commuted to work up a very steep, single-file pathway round the back of some hill-side terraced housing, a mountain-bike descended towards me, horrendously out of control. The rider saw me late and must have skidded five metres in his efforts to avoid me. I veered off into some nettles as he shot narrowly past, bouncing into the verge. I was quite impressed by his riding skills but that was insanely irresponsible.

Accidents happen.

Drivers do some stupid things, so do cyclists. I'd probably say that a higher proportion of cyclists do more reckless things more frequently but it was a collision with a car that left me unconscious with 40-odd stitches needed to my face. When cars hit people, the stakes suddenly get that much higher.

MS is bad luck - so is being hit by a car - but it is not a competition and there are no prizes. At the end of life, perhaps we can compare notes and work out who was hardest done by. Until then, let's get on with it.

It's time for Lemtrada Round 2.

Chapter Eight: Lemtrada Round 2

Back to lemtrada

My second course of lemtrada is about to start in four days' time.

To bring you up to date, I was diagnosed with a degenerative neurological condition called Multiple Sclerosis ("MS") 18 months ago. Because of its aggressive progression, I opted for an aggressive treatment and had my first bout of chemotherapy treatment in October 2015. My drug of choice was lemtrada (tradename: Campath) and the recommended treatment was for a second dose 12 months later i.e. now.

It was only last week that I officially signed-up for Round 2.

Having already completed Round 1, you might have thought that this second decision was a foregone conclusion but the stakes are high so, in my anxiety, I did feel compelled to re-visit.

At the highest level, nothing has changed:

The "pros" are still based upon the analysis of large data-pools which show that, statistically, MS patients are likely to suffer fewer relapses post-lemtrada and have decelerated disability scores, both, very roughly, by a factor of 50% (MS Society).

The "cons", again, are probability-based. The "chances" of thyroid dysfunction are still 40% (MS Society); the risk of something more serious (you can't get more serious than death) are small, but not zero. More minor side-effects are much more likely, but I still take the view that, if these are short-lived, I can tolerate them if they're offset by long-term benefits.

But, drill down into the detail, and I'm another 12 months older with new concerns to fret about.

This last year has followed the same pattern as the preceding six. During the summer months I was largely in good health. Residual MS symptoms did chisel away, but they were rarely amplified beyond an ongoing background noise.

I rode my bike across the Alps.

But, scroll back to last February and March, I was laid low by a mix of a lemtrada hang-over, MS fuzziness and winter colds. The most debilitating symptom was a new one: disabling vertigo that brought me to the floor; a spinning head that kept dragging me down to my left. I started to feel badly disorientated in crowds or in noisy environments, like busy cafes or echoing rooms.

And, this October, I have, again, spent more days ill than at work. I've been suffering from a symptom I struggle to articulate, perhaps best described as a mental-fogginess or confusion (see "*Brain Fog*"). I've been finding it very difficult to work because looking at a computer screen leaves me feeling dizzy and dislocated and my cognitive function has been scrambled to the extent that when I move my cursor across a screen sometimes I can't remember why, or where it's heading. The fatigue has been bad and I can't give my body enough sleep. Right now, I'm absolutely sick of being sick.

Before my MS diagnosis, I struggled to articulate something that I knew was "wrong". Now I have been diagnosed, the above are symptoms that I want to (and *need* to) tackle with as much energy and fight as I can muster.

All this combines for an ongoing "tick" for lemtrada Round 2.

However, the biggest thing nagging away at me is the term, "elective procedure": I'm choosing to have this treatment done.

I'm choosing an illness and a hang-over that, last year, lasted five months.

I'm choosing cold-sores, body-rash, vertigo and nausea.

But, most of all, I'm choosing risk.

Despite the malaises of the mid-seasons, this summer, I was fit, healthy and happy and life was pretty much as good as it gets. MS may have been murmuring away but I was in charge.

It makes me think how gutted, *how absolutely gutted*, I would be if, by choosing this treatment, I ended up jeopardising this.

My pre-treatment appointment last week reinforced this. Since NHS certification in 2014, 20 patients have been treated at Southmead Hospital. This year, tragically, there was the first fatality. A patient died having contracted listeria in the aftermath of their infusion. To have been diagnosed with MS and to have then gone through the same difficult risk:reward decision-making process as me, only then to have been unlucky enough to be the one outlier – the one that statistically "can't be you" – makes my stomach knot in empathy, tragedy and an undirected sympathy towards a family I've never met.

This fatality does not, of course, translate to there being a 1-in-20 chance of dying at Southmead Hospital, but the news has been accompanied by the announcement that monthly blood-tests are now being advised for 10 years post-treatment, rather than just the five communicated last year. Sepsis does, however, remain an unmitigated (and unmitigat-able) risk - see the listeria that killed a patient in Bristol. The only defence offered is extremely careful guidance on post-treatment foods (no white cheese; nothing 'mouldy') and good hygiene.

And, of course, good luck.

Lemtrada Round 2: Tales from the turf

I have just finished my third day of three. Three days spent stewing in a chair, as drugs, uppers & downers, were added to my system.

Lemtrada Round 2 is now complete. As I left the Brain Centre in Southmead, blood tests were taken to confirm that my lymphocyte count was down to near-zero. *So, let the recovery commence...*

Last year, I finished my five day course, Round 1, feeling pretty beat-up. I was covered in a body-length rash with cold-sores and a grey pallor. I had black-circled eyes and a nauseous vertigo that would last for many weeks afterwards. This year, I prepared for the same.

But, so far, it turns out that my experience of Round 2 seems to be more akin to going on holiday. Perhaps I type this a bit disingenuously, to afford myself a wry smile, but I do mean this literally: the nearest physical / psychological state that I can equate this experience to has been somewhat akin to "going on a holiday", albeit a very (very) long-haul one; although do note that I'm referring only to the "going" bit, not the enjoyable bit of actually "being there".

If Day 1 was a bit like coming off a very long haul, economy class flight (reminiscent of the ones we used to make, en famille, when we lived in Australia), by the end of Day 3, the cumulative effect could be likened to getting straight back on that same plane, flying back to London - maybe stopping for a quick shower

- then returning straight back to Sydney again. I'm tired and head-achy with a sore belly, back and knees. My skin is dry and I feel a bit nauseous. My body-clock has been broken: all three nights I've been awake between 2am and 5am despite having taken sleeping pills that seem to kick-in just as my alarm sounds to wake me up. Perhaps crossing the boundary into "too much information", it's also been three days since my last bowel movement.

Maybe I need to add to my long-haul flight analogy a few hypothetical, and ill-timed, espressos from an airport bar when I was about to drop-off to sleep, then a couple of similarly ill-judged whiskey chasers from a drinks-trolley which make me feel firstly woozy and then hung-over. I've just been hit by a wave of doubt that the self-satisfaction I'm getting from this analogy is merely the drugs talking, but it even seems to hold when I consider that vertiginous dizzy feeling you sometimes get trying to take a wee in a aeroplane toilet in the middle of the night...

Some blotches have cropped up all around my neck, my whole head is pretty flushed and a shingle-like rash has appeared on my chest but these are not only painless, they are also utterly benign. So, all-in-all, although I wouldn't say I feel great, this is chemotherapy folks. Last year, I spent several hours in a foetal position trying to count the passing seconds. This year, I read books, listened to pod-casts and watched DVDs. Dare I say it, but I've felt well enough to start feeling bored. As I prepared for this stint in hospital, I researched risks and rates for thyroid issues, ITP complications, listeria and herpes infections. I didn't find any statistics for mild, but not unreasonable, levels of slight boredom. My (non-alcoholic) champagne will remain on ice for several months yet... but this feels like a relatively auspicious start.

Touch wood.

The lemtrada pebble has been dropped into the glass-pond of my life. The initial splash doesn't seem to have broken anything but the ripples have now started. The question is where they are going, how big they're going to get and at what angle they hit what shore, and when.

One month post-lemtrada Round 2: Pharmaceutification

Over the last month, I've been suffering from symptoms that have had new, usually very long, names and I've been given drugs with new, even longer names to tackle them.

It feels like the "pharmaceutification" of my body, a new, long name of my own.

The problem is that new side-effects and symptoms keep popping up as apparently discrete events, with neither rhyme, reason nor apparent pattern.

I complain about them.

Then report them.

Then the poor health care professional faced with the spaghetti-junction of a post-chemotherapy case, deals with them one-by-one, as only they can.

So far, I've been prescribed:

metoclopramide – for the nausea that was besetting me for several hours each day, like a bad hangover or seasickness;

prochlorperazine – for the debilitating vertigo which, at its worst, was pulling me so powerfully to the floor that I actually got a bump to the head as I lay down on the kitchen laminate;

omeprazole – for the intestinal cramps which hit me half an hour after food and bent me double, again, (my new party trick), on the floor;

and

gabapentin – for the swelling pins and needles in my hands, which is a familiar symptom to me, but, of late, has been painfully bad at night.

Then two days ago, my youngest son fell ill during the night. Cleaning up his sick, and washing the vomity bed sheets, cushion-covers and clothes, predictably saw me hit by a feeling of grim sickness myself.

I took him to the GP worried about his ongoing fever but the doctor took one look at my grey pallor and started examining me instead. Unusually low blood pressure and the beginnings of a throat infection apparently so he was minded to prescribe me some **penicillin** in addition to the **co-trimoxazole** that I'm already on.

Add in the **anticlovir** anti-virals that I'm still taking post treatment.

And the daily **Vitamin D** tablets.

And the regular **paracetamols** to tackle these ongoing headaches.

And this isn't where the healthcare stops.

Immediately post-lemtrada, I was told that I might be suffering from "neutropenia" because the treatment had apparently not only wiped out my lymphocytes (as intended) but had also taken out my neutrophils (not intended). So, with some parental help, I was told to rush another "urgent" blood test to Bristol...

which showed a concerning drop in my red blood cell count...

so, I did another "urgent" blood test...

...which suggested that things were not in fact that urgent but would needed another review next week.

For what it's worth, my last "urgent" blood test yesterday showed that my lymphocytes were still zero, but that nothing new was being flagged...

...apart from my "serum creatine" score, which was 550 compared to a normal, maximum of 320. This result, the doctor simply could not explain.

Oh... did I mention the **zopliclone** to help me sleep?

Or the optional extras of **tolterodine**?

I have been trying to get out of the house but have been struggling to do so.

I walked around the park.

Last weekend, I rode (more "wobbled") my bike down a cycle path but my body was so used to being in bed that I somehow managed to pull a calf muscle as I sought to register a walking pace. It was still painful the next day so I took a couple of **ibuprofen.**

Take that, body, and add those to the mix.

The problem is that the side-effects of **lemtrada** cover pretty much every medical symptom that you could imagine. And several that you probably can't.

But, of all the symptoms listed above, almost all are actually listed side-effects of **paracetamol.** And **metoclopramide**. And **prochlorperazine**. **Gabapentin** and **ibuprofen** too. As a result, all these drugs, however well intended, feel as though they're making things even more messy.

Maybe the doctors should just be looking me in the eyes and telling me to toughen up but it would take a brave health care practitioner to do that. For them, prescribing another box of pills is probably the safe option and could never be described as being negligent. So maybe I should just be toughening up all by myself? As this MS condition goes on, I realise more and more that its treatment has to be self-managed to some degree. Each consultation with a doctor becomes an act of drama with two participants rather than just a one-way discussion with a professional; no one can know “your MS” better than you.

Right now, I want to get these drugs out of my system, get back to work... and get back on my bike.

Two months post-lemtrada Round 2

My in-laws came to visit last weekend. And nephews, uncles, aunties and all. I never thought I'd be the adult saying this but, my goodness, those kids really do grow fast. *"I remember when you were just this tall..."* Toddlers become boys become teenagers, in what seems like the blink of an eye.

As the building work still going on in our house continues at what feels like glacial pace, removed observers occasionally pop round *"amazed at all the change... " "can't believe how much has been done..."*

Our friend nearby has just had her baby. *"No way! That's been nine months already??!"*

This last week, I rode my bike again. And got myself into work.

I heard, *"I can't believe you're back so soon!" "You're so brave to be back on the bike!"* For me, however, it's been a very long seven weeks... and, although the trees must now be thinner, I don't yet feel out of the woods.

Tiredness, fatigue and indeed pain, are so subjective. My experiences of A&E, being asked to grade my own pain between 1-10 immediately prompts the thought that I could be anywhere on that scale depending upon who is asking and why... but, right now, I feel like my batteries are seriously low whoever is doing the asking. Kind comments like *"I can't believe you're back so soon..." "You're so strong back on the bike!"* tempt me to retort with how far from easy I'm finding this recovery process.

Yesterday morning, I briefly rode my bike alongside some friends in Bristol. It was a beautiful, blue sky, winter's day. *"...back on the bike!"*

Yesterday afternoon, I was phoned by my neurological consultant to discuss my latest blood results. My lymphocytes (which my treatment was designed to target) were still almost zero. My neutrophils (another element of the body's immune response) were still considerably lower than normal and fall within the boundaries of a condition called "neutropenia". Neither had moved in seven weeks. As a result, and perhaps most pertinently to the phone call, my overall white blood cell count had fallen a further 50% since the reading taken immediately post-treatment (my overall figure is now two compared to a healthy range of 4-11). All this information can probably be summarised as: yes, I may be back on the bike; but I'm still cycling in the woods, not yet through them. The consultant encouraged me to continue to take things easy and to perhaps avoid work and its germs for a bit longer. I pointed out that, at home, both my boys had been pretty ill last week, off school with coughs, colds, sickness, headaches and vomiting...

Vulnerable to infection, sleeping 10 hours a night, but also *"Back so soon!"* and *"Strong on the bike!"*. Health, like A&E pain, would seem to be in the eye of the beholder. I hear of lemtrada patients who returned to full-time work a fortnight after their treatment and wonder what they would give their "fatigue score" and, perhaps more interestingly, I wonder that they would report if they were me? How do they cope when their vision starts swimming and they need to lie down when they're mid-task? Are they just made of sterner stuff?

Happy Christmas

Out on a bike ride last week, one of my companions lamented (/laughed) at the phone-calls received from his son, who is away at university. These calls come out of the blue and start with teenaged charm turned to the max. After the pleasantries though, the request for a little financial help is never slow to follow and, of course, the love/curse of a parent is to succumb.

Poor parents, always reached for in times of need. I'm probably guilty of calling mine most typically when one of my boys (or me!) are ill – *"What medical emergency is it this time?"* It is usually when I'm most seething with frustrations at my MS that I'm sufficiently exercised into writing a blog. I have wondered if this is just my own way, subconsciously, of reaching out for support... *"O pity me!"*

So what disaster is it this time?

59 days post-lemtrada and I've just been out on my bike.

I wheezed on the hills but for the first time in ages, I felt strong. This mild excuse of a winter's day had blue skies and not a breath of wind. On one of the longest steady descents I reached forward onto the drop bars and pushed my highest gear. I stood on my pedals coming around the corner on newly-laid tarmac and raced to the next bend. My malaises seemed to melt away.

I've ridden 12,000 miles this calendar year but few have given me as much pleasure.

After all the professional turbulence of the last few weeks, and uncertainty, a previous client has just offered me a new contract for next year. As a contractor, I rarely get feedback (unless it's criticism!) so a repeat contract is probably as near as I'll ever come to, if not praise, at least some level of acceptance. And it provides a financial breath of relief.

The building work, which has been going on in our house for over 15 months now, is coming to an end. The damage caused by a burst water pipe a fortnight ago has been decorated away. As I type, a painter is putting the finishing touches to our new, white gloss door frames.

A couple of weeks ago, our car was written-off, "T-boned" side-on by an errant driver. We then enjoyed the stresses of a front wheel blow-out and the delights of filling our diesel engine with £65 of petrol...

...but my wife has just successfully navigated a week of smooth commuting in her replacement vehicle without so much as a parking ticket (*at least, not one she's admitted to!)*

Our Christmas tree stands, freshly decorated, ready for the weekend to come.

My five year old, has penned his letter to Santa with a dedicated focus that brought a tear to my eye. He spent his nativity play, back to the audience, showing impressive stoicism as he tried to attach his King's cape, which seemed to have a life of its own.

For his part, my nine year old, had atop his own Christmas List: "More Independence." In case the point wasn't made, this was swiftly followed by: "More Freedom." So the teenage years approach...

I sit at my desk drinking a fresh, strong coffee. I look out the window at our garden and ponder the fact that our fencing could probably do with a clean.

A job for next year.

Happy Christmas, everyone.

Three months post-lemtrada Round 2

It's been 14 weeks since my second dose of lemtrada.

Hopefully, I'm still only on the very first rung of the long ladder of "the rest of my life" but I thought it'd be worth typing out my experiences of the last few months, not least for those who are about to embark on the same.

The similarities in the way my body reacted to Round 1 compared to Round 2 have been marked:

After both treatments, it took three weeks before I could get back to work and, even then, I had to spend a further week largely working from home. It's worth adding a footnote to this: I am self-employed so was unpaid during this time. There was certainly no reticence on my part to get back into employment, I just couldn't overcome the lethargy and spells of vertigo. As mentioned above, some patients return to work a week after their treatments but, however brave or weak you might think I am, there was no way I could have got myself back to work that soon.

After two months, the feeling of perpetual hangover seemed to fade. By then, I was doing some gentle bike rides and breathing fresh air again. At that stage, I probably could have been back at full-time work but, luckily, I was in the position of being able to slowly ramp-up through three, four then, for the first time just recently, a five day week. I am still probably working at half pace though: both my concentration and my memory seem like fuzzy relics of what they should be.

As the new year rolled into gear, slowly the side-effects of my treatment began to take a back seat. My day-to-day concerns began to focus once more upon the minutiae of getting a family routine going again. I was still taking the chance to work from home whenever possible but, on occasion, this started to become a luxury rather than a necessity.

Getting back to cycling was hard, like it always is. But by January, friends on a Saturday ride were rolling their eyes as I overtook them on climbs, "T*hought you were meant to be recovering...*" "*Easy for some!.* It hadn't felt easy though. Cold, dark mornings wrapped up in thermal gear, trying to get my body going again, when it didn't really want to. It was mid-January when I started to be able to accelerate up, rather than just survive, the steeper climbs. At our weekly "Lunch Club", I started to be able to do turns at the front again. Then, this last week, when my alarm sounded for those 5.30am starts, a strong coffee was enough to get me going; a month ago, it felt as though I could sleep another eight hours as my body craved more rest.

So... so far, so tentatively good.

But the neutrophils (infection-killers) in my latest blood tests are still low (0.5 compared to a healthy minimum of two) so I'm still vulnerable.

In fact, at a recent appointment at the orthopaedic department, the consultant grew concerned about apparent painful infection in my shin bone which he had heard could be linked to patients with suppressed immunity. This led to another hospital visit, another scan and another four week course of antibiotics.

Lots of letters are still pinned to my kitchen notice-board with dates and times for future hospital appointments of one sort or another. Both the NHS and I continue to keep a careful watch on my ups and downs, my readings and my scores. I have booked time-slots for monthly bloods and quarterly catch-ups as well as an umpteen referrals for this and that. It's time-consuming stuff, having MS.

But then, the kicker.

Out last Sunday morning, my optic neuritis came back. It's a really foreboding symptom and pretty debilitating. It's been 18 months since I last suffered this and, back then, it was my left eye. This time, it's definitely my right so I'm worried that this might be a new MS symptom or relapse (i.e. another lesion on the spine or brain). As I type this, I'm struggling to focus on the letters or to keep them in my gaze. I am losing track of the mouse curser when it moves across the screen.

I liked it when my day-to-day concerns had returned to the minutiae of a family routine and that my greatest stresses had become trying to fit all my appointments into a busy life. I hope this new issue with my eyesight isn't going to remind me of the bigger priorities at stake.

It's also now three weeks until March, my seasonal "MS Danger-Zone". Wondering what this might hold, I get ready to circle the wagons...

Remittance

Two years ago, my MS felt out of control.

New symptoms were appearing every few weeks and, by October 2015, my neurological consultant had accelerated me onto a course of lemtrada chemotherapy.

I had a second dose in October 2016.

It had become difficult to separate the side-effects of the drug from further MS activity but, in summary, it'd be fair to say that my health had been patchy over those intervening 12 months.

When first diagnosed, of course the hope was that my variant of the condition would be towards the less aggressive end of the scale, right at the benign end of the spectrum. This basically translates into a "relapsing-remitting" type (i.e. one that dissipates (or remits) between bouts (or relapses)).

The very best possible scenario would be that my MS actually remits entirely. There have been cases where patients diagnosed with MS have gone on to live long and healthy lives with no further interference from the condition at all, but the fact that I had already suffered so many relapses and had so many visible lesions on my brain and spine to show for them, makes this less likely.

The law of averages dictates that 85% of newly diagnosed patient in their 30s (i.e. me) will have one of those relapsing-remitting types, likely to appear, then diminish, over a period of years. But I'm afraid that the most likely overall trajectory is one of deterioration: **65%** of patients become "secondary progressive" within **10-15 years** of diagnosis. Secondary progressive means a "sustained build-up of disability" with little or no recovery between relapses.

My relationship with my MS is now one of seeking to avoid this mathematical probability, to avoid the occurrence of relapses and to rejoice as much as possible in the fact that I'm not there yet. *And, of course, fingers crossed, might never be.*

Right now, at the beginning of summer 2017, my MS symptoms are no more than murmurs, and I'm recovering from the minor bugs of everyday life within normal timeframes, rather than suffering from them for weeks at a time.

Statistically, this is probably no more than where I should be: a period of remittance in-between relapses. But I can't help but be more optimistic than that: I've now got two bouts of chemotherapy under my belt and have now been adhering to a much healthier regimes of MS-Diet and careful sleep patterns for over two years. Although I remain mindful of the false dawns of hope, I can't deny myself the excitement of feeling so very improved:

- I would judge that I have been as healthy as I can remember for perhaps eight or nine years.
- I am pushing niggles to the side and I've been out cycling, working full-time, painting garden fences and mowing the lawn. All things I have stopped taking for granted.
- I'm lining up big cycling plans for the summer and have been getting myself ready, body and bike, for adventures to come.

I gritted my teeth when a stress fracture in my right foot took six weeks to heal and I continue to do so now with a different issue in my right knee. Frustratingly, the pain there is being caused by a titanium pin inserted there many years ago. The surgeon is reluctant to do anything whilst my post-chemo immune system remains low: my latest blood results still show my lymphocytes struggling at 0.5 against a normal minimum of two.

So, I ignore my arthritis, cope with my grumbling optical neuritis and aim my bike at the horizon. As fast as I can.

65%. 10-15 years.

I chase more time. I chase life, perhaps always thinking that I might find it at the top of the next hill.

I feel pretty tired today but I'm planning a quick spin at lunch.

Despite the drizzling rain, I don't want to risk missing it.

One barometer of my MS that I reflect on, is the scope of my "future gaze": whether I have the capacity to look at future months & years or I am just focussing on the next day. Everyone will empathise with how your world view and forethoughts shrink during periods of stress or illness; I'd have thought that everyone with children will empathise with that sensation of just trying to get through each day, juggling water and herding cats.

To some extent, I have been living in week-long blocks for the last couple of years. I've been making plans for each weekend but being more tentative on a grander scale. My confidence had been severely dented when I thought I'd have to drop out of the long planned Alpine Cycling trip described above (see "*Pre-ride. On the brink of something*"). This had meant letting a friend down at the very last minute as I struggled to work out what was going on with some grumbling MS symptoms. I was finding that pre-planned weekends were proving to be the source of anxiety, rather than excitement. But this year, I do think that things are definitely evolving (for the better). I've been booking summer holidays, both en famille and solo and have, somewhat cagily, been letting my optimism grow. Over the next fortnight, I'll be dipping my toes back into the water of a night out in London, and a weekend playing golf with some old friends; although I approach these MS-tests with trepidation, there is also the definite emergence of a new confidence.

Reading between the lines above, you'll see that I'm have been feeling pretty good regarding the various challenges of my MS. This has been one of those periods in time that I have been holding my breath waiting for....

...so – to use what I believe is the technical term – I cycled the hell out of Spring.

I raced up a hill or two with my friends at "Lunch Club"; made new friends climbing up to the ridge and viewpoints of the White Horse above Avebury; did a 200 mile ride up to the Heart of England (and beyond); and enjoyed a weekend away in the stunning hills of Southern France. These latter two days certainly hit the cycling sweet-spot: a friend and I toured the Gorge du Verdon upon roads that clung to precipitous cliffs and hair-pinned through tunnels and caves, up to ski-resorts and mountain-top espresso-stops and down to cobbled French villages where we filled our water bottles in age-old fountains. We even fitted in a "gastronomic" seven-course dinner in our remote overnight stop-over. Our ravenous 200km-cycled appetites were given a lesson in patience as 'amuse-bouche' followed one bite-size course after another. *"Encore du pain, s'il vous plait?!!"*

Ageing, arthritic and MS, I can't just click my fingers and do weekends like that anymore. It involved 400km of cycling, 30,000 feet of climbing and, therefore, having some serious base miles under my belt. These adventures were the archetypal "summer smiles" earned by "winter miles". These rewards don't always come easily: a couple of months earlier, I had been in Southmead hospital (again) discussing the stress fracture in my right metatarsal, probably caused by some over-training. Talk was of the need for a month's rest. I contemplated this... before then cycling home.

Another little hurdle.

But – let me check – my "future gaze" barometer still reads well. My thoughts and ambitions are still upwardly looking at the summer and beyond.

If this is remittance, then roll on.

Not remittance

For a couple of months, things were indeed pretty rosy. I'd been back at work, full time. I'd been riding more and more miles on my bike and describing how I felt with tentative optimism.

Then, all of a sudden, last weekend, MS was back, whipped up from these benign conditions like a prairie storm. Snarling, snapping and biting... yanking furiously at its tether, spitting and evil, fangs bared and razor-sharp claws unsheathed. I'd forgotten that it packed such a mean ferocity.

The outlook of blue skies had briefly showed the smallest hint of a warning sign, a minor head cold, before – *bang!* – a flare-up was upon me before I'd had time to suspect it.

It seemed to affect my left-hand side the worst. My wife and I looked at my strangely curled/dropped left foot which I could no longer straighten, my left hand became all clumsy and fumbling and the buzz of pins and needles burst into something much more angry down both legs and arms. I was also worried that the focus in my eyes seemed to be confused again but, thankfully this symptom was short-lived, disappearing after one good night's sleep.

MS was reminding me, a click of its fingers is all it takes. Once again, I felt weak to its power, on my knees to its strength, as it selected which symptoms to activate from its own pick'n'mix sweetshop.

Exasperated. Angry. Upset... tired.

Growing hope that my lemtrada treatment might be putting off these flare-ups now seemed misguided.

MS, my savage friend, needs once again to be calmed back down. Maybe he's striking out in fear, like a panicked and wounded animal, but maybe he's just a symptom of my mis-firing immune system and feels no more fear than a comet in the sky or pebble on a beach.

I ask to be given strength but feel bowed, not broken. MS certainly is a mean task-master but when this episide is over, I am going to get out on my bike and put him back in his box.

I don't want to stop coming back for more... *MS, you hide in the shadows; I'm staying here in the light.*

Update*: Despite the melodrama above, that bout only lasted a bit more than a week. Of course, the benefit of hindsight would have made the event so much less upsetting because, arguably, the worst symptom that goes hand-in-hand with any perceived MS-activity, is that of fear. This is the fear of longer-term damage and the fear of being only at the start of one of those never-ending bouts which make me feel so down.*

Chapter Nine:
The rest of life

Hill reps and an Everesting

I'm making cycling plans for later this summer, some serious undertakings for adventure. I'm planning to do what I love doing: getting out on my bike and travelling to new places, on new roads, through new landscapes.

I know, however, that I can't just pursue these dreams on a whim. Preparation will be all: logistics; equipment and, of course, body. "Preparation", then very much keeping my fingers crossed that my MS remains locked in its box.

Of course, in many ways, cycle-touring is what I've already spent years gearing up for. I've commuted by bike, entered events which have dangled goals just beyond my easy reach and have long sought to explore new roads and find new hills, be it on my own or out with clubs or friends. But the time is now nigh to train specifically for this summer's miles, uncertain weathers and rugged terrains. I need to get ready to ride with the inevitability of the unexpected so, to this end, I've been doing more and more "hill reps" which basically means finding some hills... then riding up them, on repeat.

As any cyclist will attest, this can be a tough medicine, but I'm of the opinion that every such obstacle surmounted now, will stand me in better stead for the future.

On the 23rd June, I started early on my bike. It was nigh on the summer solstice. Even at 5am, it was already uncommonly hot. The previous, truncated night I'd spent tossing and turning beside the biggest fan I could find.

Because I wasn't planning to venture far from home, my bike was as light as it could be: race wheels; new tyres; and even a cleaned cassette. I was in shorts and a T-shirt. If I was to be climbing hills, I couldn't have done it any lighter.

I sought out a local climb called Bannerdown… then rode up it. I rode up it, paused for breath, then turned around and descended back to the start again.

The pain I'd been having with my right foot had gone. I had only the merest hint of MS pins and needles.

I felt good and rode up it again. Rep number two.

Repeated ascents then began to tick past. Two became four, then five. Slowly I began to lose count amongst my water breaks and stops for food.

Rep by rep, however, the temperature was also slowly rising… and rising. It hit 20 degrees when it was still early morning.

I tried to drink as much as I could because I soon realised that dehydration would become my biggest impediment. The drip-drip of my sweat soon became a flow and salt began to sting my eyes. My pauses at the summits became longer and my recovery breathing deeper.

I knew I wasn't drinking enough but couldn't manage to get more liquid down.

The thermometer reached 33 degrees.

Tiredness began to creep in. Firstly, my calves, then twinges of cramp in my thigh. The pressure points on the balls of my feet and palms of my hands began to hurt in the heat. I was beginning to get a dehydration headache, but chose to carry on. I had decided to ride until I had nothing left to give, for no reason other than to see where I could get to. It didn't scare me.

Another ascent to the same summit. Back to the same starting point again. *The Grand Old Duke of York*.

I recalled a memory from my childhood when my mother would read me a book of fairy tales ("Fairy Tales and Fantastic Stories"). I always found them unduly spooky and a bit unsettling before bed but couldn't help but be enticed by their sensation of eeriness.

As I started another climb, I remembered a tale about a goblin, who was trying to tempt a young girl to the magical Goblin City:

Short or long to Goblin City?
The straight way's short
But the long way's pretty

I found the image of the goblin unnerving, as was the beat of this repeated rhyme.

As it turned out, the girl was so beset by indecision over this choice that the tale ended abruptly with her opportunity removed.

I turned back down the hill again.

Back to the start.

The long way around.

If I had been her, I would have chosen the long, pretty way.

A straight-line through life would feel no more than a race to the end. Without the hill reps.

I was getting more and more tired as I rode back up again.

I had known as long ago as sunrise that the heat of the day would be my biggest challenge but I was struggling to counter it. By late afternoon, I was beginning to feel so dehydrated that I began to wonder if I might be dangerously so. I had drunk eight litres of water and hadn’t gone to the loo once. It still hadn't been enough. My efforts began to feel as though they were almost done.

Although I was low on energy, I stopped being able to get food down. I tried sucking on some boiled sweets but had to spit them out as my body refused even those. I began to feel pretty sick.

What was this all about? This was me, setting the bar for my summer, putting down a building block, seeing where I was and where I could go.

Eventually, I stopped my bike for the final time. My right hand was starting to cramp up on the brake levers.

I was supremely tired.

I had done 8,950 metres of climbing, slightly more than the height of Mount Everest.

When I got home, I lay down and both my legs started pulsing with cramp. But nothing could stop me drifting off into the deepest of sleeps.

The long way around indeed. And, like life, certainly not a straight line.

I'm really happy for that to be my choice.

La Maratona

Two years ago, I rode a bike event called “L'Etape”, a hilly, mountainous day-race plagiarised from the Tour de France. In the week leading up to it, my MS had been rumbling away with rising menace, and on the day itself, I had somewhat disintegrated on the bike, beset by cramps and issues with my eyesight. It occurred to me then that I might not ever ride a similar event again. Maybe this was something that I was going to have to surrender to MS. Certainly I still recall most vividly those sensations of body malfunction, clear mental scars that beg future caution.

As I type the above, I consider again how far I feel as though I have come since that day for, last week, I rode “La Maratona”. This is an event of similarly challenging parcours, this time in the Dolomites rather than the Alps. The total climbing was going to be more and the hills were going to be steeper.

I may not have “raced” the course, I paced it more akin to a sociable audax, but I did complete it. My MS did briefly raise its head above the parapet but with barely a whimper rather than a battle-cry.

The Event

Road cycling can be a sport so beautifully pure in its simplicity: get on a bike. Ride it.

But, because one of its pleasures is experience of landscape, I often lift-up the whole process, just so I can drop it down again into vistas anew: of late, Wales; the Cairngorms; and, on a few memorable occasions, the Alps.

Entering “events”, especially abroad, is another matter again. It feels as though you’re transporting the whole circus of bike, bike bag and equipment. It's like moving home for one brief weekend of riding.

Getting to the Dolomites was this to an extreme. Our party of five converged from our far-flung homes via plane and car with disassembled equipment, wardrobes of kit (“for every season”), bags of energy gels, bars and pills, suncreams and gloves.

We checked into an apartment and ate pizza at the nearest restaurant we could find.

We spent hours building our bikes back up again from flat-pack, testing brakes, gears and re-inflating tyres.

Registering for the event entailed an hour-long queue amongst hoards of fellow cyclists. It meant copies of passports, doctor’s certificates and insurance forms.

All this just to ride a bike.

The travel, queuing and stresses were exhausting, MS or not. My friends must have been mystified as I slept over 10 hours on both the first two nights.

On the morning of the event, our alarms went off at 4am (yes... FOUR am!) but, when we got to the start, we were far from early and had to join the massed ranks of other queuing cyclists shivering in the pre-dawn cold. I was underdressed. Veterans around us donned winter jackets and beanies. My limbs and muscles felt a bit washed up and tired.

When the ride did slowly crank into action, my core felt cold but the roads were too busy to get up any pace or rhythm. The first climb was clogged with cyclists, many tutting at the frustrations of slow progress. At several hairpin bends, an approaching wave of clicking sounds washed down the road towards me, cyclist after cyclist clipping out of their cleats as they came to a congested standstill.

By the time I reached the first summit and started to descend I was still grumpy with cold. The downhill had to be ridden with the hand-brake on as swarms of bikes edged and wobbled round the sharp bends. On one high-speed turn I locked my rear wheel as I broke to avoid the clutter.

The dark skies were threatening rain. *God forbid*. I was already wearing every garment and any rain would have pushed me over the edge. With surprising clarity of logic, I realised that if it did start to rain I would have to give up immediately.

Upon completion of the initial circuit, a large number of riders left the road onto the shorter course and the tarmac freed up. At last, I developed a rhythm on my pedals and my body warmed up. Bit by bit, my muscle aches began to loosen and the temperatures started lifting; I even rolled down my arm warmers on the ascents. The next downhill was an exhilarating pleasure and my grumpiness began to melt away into smiles.

Rather than slaloming between a forest of bikes, I began to look up and soak in the views: stunning valley-scapes and vertical outcrops of rock. Local residents came out to support and rang colossal cow bells as we passed. I fell into amiable conversation with a young lad from Dublin who was riding at the same pace as me.

Some 80km in, I hadn't needed a food-stop and had the two largest climbs still to go. It was difficult to gauge how much energy I had initially burned just to stay warm, set against how much energy I'd saved by riding relatively slowly for the first hour or so. I decided to gamble and to hit Passo Giau, the penultimate climb, without further provisions. Little did I know what an absolute beast of an ascent it would prove to be.

After the first few kilometres of steepness, I grew more and more convinced that it was about to flatten out (it had to?) but, if anything, it reared up even more. I could no longer hide from the fact that I was going to run empty; the dreaded cyclist's "bonk" when the body's fuel dramatically runs out. It hit me with about 3km of the climb still to go and those last 3,000m were ridden through desperately gritted teeth at barely walking pace. My new friend from Dublin overtook me again and, after a brief chat, kindly handed me an energy gel and joked that he wouldn't be impressed if I overtook him again before the top.

At the summit's food stop, I drank a litre of coke and sparked up as though I'd be given a shot of adrenalin to the heart.

I hurtled down the last descents and rode the last long climb, and the final, short one, at, what was for me, race pace.

I effectively time-trialled the last 20km and finished with a sprint alongside a couple of other riders as we lunged for the line... fighting for 1,423rd place.

Upon finishing, my body coursed with endorphins and I was buzzing. Over the last few miles I had asked my legs, again and again, for more and they'd been able to provide. I had felt strong and capable.

I was so invigorated that I could barely sleep that night with flushes of excitement, caffeine and sugar-highs.

That, I realised, is why they do it. Those crazy cyclists who transport their lives to the Dolomites just to go on a bike ride.

It can make you feel so alive.

After the long, long journey back home my back ached. So too did my knees. And shoulders. And muscles and bones.

As I unpacked my bike from its box, I discovered that the rear derailleur (the thing that shifts the bike's gears) had snapped off in transit.

They're not easy, these so-called events. This so-called life.

But if you don't do such things, your life would just be a straight-line... I quite like the bumps, and the hills.

Why? North-West Scotland

Why?

I've spent the last few days cycling around northern Scotland.

I dipped my toes in the North Sea on one side and into the Atlantic on the other.

At times, the road across to Lochinver felt as if it were on the moon: remote, desolate and windswept. At others, it blurred into a water-coloured and washed-out landscape dripping with drizzle and mists. The wind blew on and on; even when I fell asleep at night it still echoed in my ears and in my dreams.

And the skies were of every conceivable colour, all at once. From one single viewpoint, I could see greys, blues, whites and blacks and every combination in between. Parts of the landscape were bathed in sunlight whilst, way off in the distance, I could see what looked like heavy rain.

It felt good for the soul.

To a cyclist long-used to the pottering, enclosed country lanes around the Cotswolds, the scale of the Scottish landscapes were pretty breath-taking in grandeur. Mountains, lochs, coastal inlets and isles disappeared to the horizon.

These roads have existed for centuries but an interesting phenomenon has taken place over just the last couple of years as they have been packaged up and sold as a product ready for tourist consumption: "The North Coast 500". Designed to boost the remote area's economy, these beautiful roads have been given a name, T-shirts and memorabilia have been put on sale, and sign-posts have appeared reminding foreign visitors not to drive on the right. In this way, this landscape, that isn't owned, has somehow been boxed up and gift-wrapped for the hoards and the impact has been remarkable.

All the locals I spoke to reported an enormous growth in visitor numbers and I was overtaken by a procession of foreign number plates: French cars and German, Dutch & Danish campervans.

When I stopped at picnic sites, I overheard families chit-chatting in Italian and tour-guides calling out in one, two, then three, different languages. The hosts I spoke to, however, seemed a bit begrudging of this boost as their roads crowded up and their litter bins filled to overflowing. Even the hostel-owner I spoke to lamented that they were now fully booked all the time (*oh no!*)

Whilst acknowledging that this was peak season, some bottlenecks did feel at capacity and some drivers' patience with cyclists was wearing a bit thin.

"Why don't you get a feckin' car?!"

And, the slightly more constructive,

"Turn your feckin' lights on!"

(I preferred the, "Go! Go! You crazy cyclist!")

Cars drove from one designated viewpoint to the next. Coaches followed.

The hassle of disembarking proved too much for some. I saw one couple stop in the middle of the road as the driver filmed from his seat and his passenger leant fully out of the window to take a photo.

Coinciding my arrival at one spot with a coach-load of snappers, I tentatively asked a rather rotund, friendly looking man if he'd mind please taking a photo of me,

"No, no, I'm not at work now."

His "North Coast 500" T-shirt, replete with bus logo, barely covered his sitting-in-a-coach-for-500-miles belly.

Luckily the area I covered was large enough so that much of the time I felt removed from the busy world. At one point, I came to a stop because a cluster of four stags were blocking the road barely ten metres in front of me. We eyed each other nervously for a minute or so before they slowly walked off and into the trees.

On my second night, I ended up cycling almost 30 miles to find anywhere that would sell me anything that I could eat for dinner. This turned out to be a can of bean-hash and a bag of Scottish teacakes that had gone out of date yesterday.

And, the next morning, pretty hungry, I rode for over three hours before I eventually found an open cafe. At 10am, I was the only, rather bedraggled, customer.

"Hi. I could *really* do with a hot drink please."

"Hmmmm." The hostess looked hesitant.

"We are booked up for lunch."

The neatly laid tables all had notes reserving themselves for the next coach party at midday.

I managed to twist her arm into a quick 10-minute window for a coffee and soup.

If the first two-thirds of the trip were the joyous pleasure of a new landscape explored, the last leg was more of a battle as I was buffeted by wind and rain.

My right knee was hurting (and neck and back and metatarsal) and I was having to adjust my pedal strokes accordingly. I was feeling far from my best.

Increasingly thirsty, hungry and getting a few shivers I wondered whether my snood, which was now wet, was shielding me from cold, or just exacerbating it.

Ruminations and concerns of earlier in the ride – mortgages, jobs & healthcare – had dissipated away and I was left with the basics of needing food and drink and riding back towards my love for my family.

The motion of cycling does mean that, when all else is stripped away, what really matters can step to the fore with an overwhelming clarity. I was thinking of my children.

I considered how I must keep this perspective when I get home.

Maybe this isn't "The Why" but it feels like something important, worth writing about.

Love. Life. Wind on my back, rain in my face and fresh, clean air.

The glorious North Coast 500. *Or 350 miles of it anyway.*

To ride every road
The Coast of Wales 500

The website Strava can generate "heatmaps", visual summaries of every road you've ever ridden.

For me, immediately around my house and work, almost every road is painted in red. Then, as the map expands, these red lines spread out and the cluster of colour dissolves into thinner and thinner tendrils of exploration, until they, too, turn back to whence they came.

There are other epicentres of activity around my other cycling-haunts: North London, the Cairngorms and even the Alps. Red lines of memories which serve as my photo albums and diary.

I've started to look at these maps as I plan my next rides in order to fill in missing roads and find new ones.

On a recent ride with my local cycling pals, I got excited about a new left turn and announced my goal: "to cycle every road."

"What? 'Every road' where? In the Cotswolds?"

"No, no, my friend... in the world."

Much still to do.

Last week I did a multi-day ride around the coastal perimeter of Wales.

Although coastal cycling is exposed, and often with tough gradients, it can certainly rivals mountain ranges for dramatic scenery.

I started in the south-eastern corner, crossing into Wales via the Severn Bridge, before passing along the South Welsh Riviera (the industrial conurbations of Port Talbot and Cardiff); through the summer holiday crowds around the Gower and St Davids; then up, north, along quieter and more rugged roads towards Snowdonia. The north-west had a much flatter profile, sweeping along a floodplain all the way up to the Isle of Anglesey. Having gone all that way, I insisted on doing a loop of that island before heading east, back across the top of the principality to Chester train station and a much faster (and motorised!) journey home.

Initially, my route across the South of Wales felt a bit constricted.

The roads were busy with chains of holiday traffic and every town was beset by traffic lights and queues at the coffee shops. All the cars seemed to want to be somewhere else and were intent on getting there in a hurry.

I largely stuck to minor roads but kept accidentally finding myself on dual carriageways where I felt obliged to cycle as fast as my legs could carry me to get away from the revs of impatient drivers.

I took photos of smokestacks, steelworks and industrial recycling centres. These cycling-badlands were the same roads where I've had to swerve to avoid a dead horse and had bricks thrown at me whilst a group of kids shouted, "Go Forest!" *(which, I guess, is pretty funny...)*

Cardiff Bay offered a bit more sheen with its fancy Assembly Building, boardwalks and tidal barrier but the first real beach I came to was Swansea, where misty rain was herding the tourists into steamy tearooms. Tenby also had a beautiful beach but the town was bursting at the seams with visitors. It was only when I got to Pembroke, turned the corner and started heading north, that the landscape really started to open up.

In the morning on my second day, the sunshine was desperately trying to burn through and succeeded enough so that the beaches started to dot with multi-coloured bathers for my obligatory photos. Riding alongside the tourist railway at Aberdovey was a real highlight and, by then, the sea was glittering.

A hint of a tailwind and even my route miscalculations started doing me favours: a wrong turn near Barmouth meant that I had to catch a speedboat across the river whilst a gaggle of fascinated children asked me about my mysterious tri-bars and lycra.

By the time I crossed the Menai Bridge into Anglesey, I had started to curse the buffeting cross-winds a bit but I was still where I wanted to be, in the great outdoors, feeling a very long way from an office desk. The road came to an end in Holyhead and I could go no further north.

Heading back to the east along the top of Wales took me along a remarkable web of interconnected cycle-ways. They bobbed and weaved up, down, over and around the coastal road. At times, ocean spray dowsed my bike and windblown sand threatened wheel-spinning skids. I was tired after a few long days of riding but a steady drip-drip of beautiful photo opportunities kept me enthused: Llandudno castle, the oceanic wind farms out at sea, the spiky coastal defences at Penmaenmawr and the occasional tourist honey-pot of a pleasure beach. For lunch, I sat with my feet dangling in the huge seafront paddling pool at Llandudno, feeling quite as happy can be.

For the last 20km, I rode on the extraordinary "concrete beach" past Rhyl. The camber of this storm defence pulled me towards the surf of high tide. I wobbled a bit uncertainly in the gusty winds and rode very cagily as I overtook the many dog walkers. It began to feel like a good time to turn off whilst I was still upright. I could see England way off in the distance.

I stayed the last night of my tour with my sister's in-laws.

I arrived pretty roughed up by the weather and pretty tired.

The dad laughed, "I can't believe you've done all that in three days – it'd take me that long to drive it!"

I was fed a delicious dinner.

As I looked in the mirror before bed I thought how tired I looked. My hands were buzzing with pins and needles. They were in my left cheek and neck too, which has become a new symptom of late. My arthritic knee felt particularly stiff and sore.

I am very much looking forward to a nice new, circular red line on my "heatmap". This one was hard-earned.

Planning

This week I fly to Portland, Oregon.

I'm planning to cycle the Pacific Way, down the West Coast of the USA.

This has been a trip over a decade in the making since I first sketched out a route and added it to my bucket list.

More recently, it has been eight months in the planning during which time I've booked flights, bought kit... and cycled over 10,000 miles in preparation.

It'll be a testing tour and will involve cycling some long distances over some varied terrain, probably through some varied weather conditions.

I hope I'm ready for it.

And, yes, I hope it'll be fun.

The first time I ever really rode a bike was 20 years ago.

A Raleigh Pioneer bought for £195.

I bought it not to commute, nor to pop down to the shops (for which it was probably built), but to cycle from Lands End to John O'Groats, some 1,200 miles.

Never having ridden more than five miles at once I wasn't sure how long this might take – the local bike shop suggested perhaps 60 miles a day – so, being a young man, I planned on nearer a hundred, booked a train ticket to Truro and photocopied about

40 pages of my Granny's Road Atlas of the UK to stuff into my back-pack.

I wore my running shoes, gym vest and tracksuit trousers and packed my bobble hat and golfing-waterproofs in case of rain.

On Day 1, I bought a five-pack of Mars bars in case I needed boosts of energy along the way.

I didn't pack a spare inner tube, nor a puncture repair kit. I didn't even know that you could get punctures on a bicycle, let alone how to change a tyre.

This year, I mull over which of my wheels, and tyres, to take. Given that most of the route is likely to be on decent surfaces – albeit with the likelihood of rain – I opt for my lighter, "race" wheels coupled with winter tyres which are more puncture resistant and offer greater grip should the roads get slippery. I do worry that a broken spoke on this option would present a significantly greater problem but, on balance, I figure I'd be unlucky if that happened.

I've downloaded my route into my handheld GPS unit and I've packed a spare.

20 years ago, on my second day of riding, I started to feel dizzy with hunger and tiredness.

I had arrived at my first night's hostel well after sunset and had eaten only a simple dinner of boiled pasta.

Mid-morning, barely 20 miles into the day, my bike had wobbled ono the verge of the road and I had laid down on the ground, unable to carry on. Eventually I found my way to a pub, waited for it to open, and then ordered two lunches and a pint of coke.

I hadn't realised how hard this "holiday" of mine might be. By the end of Day 3, pretty much the whole of my backside was red-raw with saddle-soreness. I stopped at a chemists and bought an industrial tub of Vaseline. It dawned on me that cycling with cotton boxer shorts was a bad idea so experimented with going "commando" instead which was no better.

That night, in Tiverton, my hands were so numb from their unfamiliar position of the day that I couldn't hold my cutlery at dinner and ended up having to shovel in my pasta with a great deal of slurping.

But, despite all this, the trip was beginning to feel like a proper adventure. I was learning every minute... and was excited about what I was doing.

The close-knit, patchwork fields of Devon and Cornwall, with their sharp, twisty climbs and tall hedges, slowly gave way to a less confined landscape as I rode up the Welsh borders.

I was learning what and how to eat more sensibly and how often I needed to stop and rest.

I made my way through the industrial (ex-industrial) heartlands of the Midlands – through towns I had previously only known through their famous football teams – and, by the time heavy rains were pouring through Northern England and the Lake District, I was on a high. I had almost ridden the length of England and I was no longer just surviving, I was enjoying

My arm- and leg-warmers are lightweight and flexible enough for changing weather conditions. I'm going to pack a couple of protein bars and energy gels should I be caught short.

Through much trial and error, I've lately been wearing my "Ale" shorts for long rides. Combined with ASSOS chamois cream they're as good a way as I've found to avoid chaffing. Although they're expensive, I long-ago decided that they were worth the investment given the amount of cycling I do.

It was only when I was half-way up Scotland that I dared to think that I might actually get the whole way to John O'Groats. Suddenly it began to seem actually within range.

But my bike was beginning to really creak and grind. The incessant rain, which had lasted a few days, and associated road-grit, felt as they were bringing me to a standstill. I stopped in a lay-by for shelter and saw that my chain was almost wholly brown with rust and was almost locked to my touch.

By happenstance, at that moment a farmer appeared out of the rain on his tractor. I showed him my issue and, by way of a prompt can-do response, he opened up an oil can and doused the whole of my bike in thick engine oil before rubbing it in with a cloth. He asked where I was heading, and when I told him, he laughed uproariously before driving off, leaving me to the stench of diesel.

This year, I've packed a miniature bottle of bike oil. Each night I'll be cleaning my bike, re-indexing my gears and adjusting my brakes. As well as a pump, I'll pack a few CO2 canisters to ensure I can get my tyres up to adequate pressure.

I worry again about my choice to go with my lighter, less robust wheels.

When I got to John O'Groats it left like something of an anti-climax. I was alone and it was still raining.

However, as I turned back towards my hostel for the night a small cluster of other cyclists pulled in. They were proper cyclists with road bikes, lycra... and probably their own spare inner tubes. Then I recognised them – I'd seen them many days before near the Scottish Border. They seemed genuinely delighted to see me,

"No way!"

"I can't believe you made it!"

"We never thought you would!"

"The man in the bobble hat!"

For the first time, cycling offered some sense of pride too.

I think back to me, 20 years ago.

I knew then that, through sheer youthful exuberance, I had managed to force a square peg through a round hole and cycle the length of the country.

That night, I had celebrated with youthful exuberance and drunk (much too much) whisky in the nearest Scottish pub.

On my return journey back south, I had met up with an old friend in Edinburgh and, through sheer youthful exuberance, we had stayed up all night drinking (much too much) whisky in all the Scottish pubs we could find.

Now not so youthful, and perhaps not so much exuberance, but the lure of life still feels as strong as ever.

These last few months? They have been training for me. Training for my trip to the USA to come. All roads have been leading to here.

Time, if ever it were needed, for my MS to stay in its box.

The Pacific Coast: a travelogue

To some extent, America is a known quantity to us Brits.

My sense of the country has long been channelled by films and TV so, to some degree, I knew what to expect when I arrived in Portland Airport.

From my first step through US Customs (warmly welcomed by a US cop, complete with gun holster and sparkling policeman's badge) to the sight of the Hollywood letter-boards (as I rolled into LA), this whole trip was to be a satisfying tick-box exercise of all that I imagined the US to be. One by one I was seeing the real versions of all those screen-based myths.

My arrival in Oregon kick-started this theory as "Portlandia" (the TV myth) seemed to be the perfect embodiment of the Portland for real, or vice versa. Tattooed hipsters served me coffee, gave me cycling advice and offered vegan, gluten-free alternatives to every dish.

It dawned on me that I could probably have a very happy holiday just chilling out in that one city... but quitting my ride before I'd even started would have been the betrayal of a steady drum-roll that I had been building up for many months.

I had an adventure to get done.

On my first day, wide-eyed and fresh, I was enthused by every passing road sign, shop-front and vehicle: "Highways"; "Diner"; "Waffles"; "Pancakes"; "Gallons"; people carriers; and 4×4's.

They were the US that I already knew. It felt like I was reconnecting with an old friend.

Actually, my first day was a pretty grim route through Portland's industrial hinterland but I was far too excited to care. With a boyish excitement I was served free refills of coffee, paid small sums with big wads of single dollar bills, left tips, passed green and yellow road signs and turned right, legally, on red lights. After one, then two, visits it became clear that every diner would remind me of that early scene from Pulp Fiction.

Up-scaled

What soon became apparent was the extent to which life on the road had been so dramatically up-scaled. Rather than being squeezed onto the side of a UK road, I cycled, in what felt like relative safety, on a hard shoulder the same width as a full lane. Initially, I stuck to the main highways and, although the flow of passing traffic never abated, it passed with a cruising calmness I wasn't used to – 40-50mph, rather than with a roaring acceleration nearer to 70. The theme of this "up-scaling" was everywhere and remained for my whole trip: from the trees, to the food portions, landscapes and people.

This was a country built upon road transportation. The highways bulldozed straight from A to B, through towns and over rivers rather than dabbling around them like they do at home. Rather than peering round one turn after another, I got used to re-orientating myself at an intersection to see my route road disappearing off to the horizon, tarmac shimmering with hazy mirages in the sun.

Up-scaled too was what I was trying to achieve. My plans demanded 250km of cycling everyday and, from the very start, I treated these distances with a nervous respect. Rather than racing breathlessly to my rest-stop each night, I cruised, rather more in keeping with the feel of the traffic, and stopped frequently, always aiming to carry more food and water than I could possibly need. I was racing no one; I was there instead to breathe in the sights.

It took me almost most 100 miles of cycling to actually get to the Pacific Coast and, even then, I smelt the sea before I saw it. One small hill later, and suddenly it was there, The Pacific Ocean, out as far as the eye could see. It would become my orientating compass for the next ten days: the huge, featureless mass to my right. Throughout my tour, a steady, inland breeze continuously drifted in from its waves.

Each variation of landscape had in common this same sense of overwhelming scale from the beaches, to the hills, farms, ranches and forests. Even the sky felt bigger as it played out its daily pattern of dawn mists followed by a steady rise in temperature to a deep afternoon blue. I wasn't used to seeing so much of it at once.

These are the images that I imagined remembering: the photogenic and the grand. Every morning with my early starts, I enjoyed the pre-dawn air, seeing first the moon and stars and then the sunrise.

However, it's a paradox of cycling touring that, at the very same time my world was growing, it was also shrinking down to the minutiae. The road surfaces ebbed and flowed and drove my moods: from the sleekest of new tarmacs that I floated over; to cracked and blistered old road coatings that had been scrunched up and wrinkled by the elements. At its worst, every passing metre jarred my bike and rattled its frame.

I wiped tiny grains of sand from my drive-train each time I passed close to a windswept beach and I eked out my small tubes of suncream and saddle-cream so that they would last the trip. It was only on my tenth, and final, day that I, at last, could use with joyous abandon whatever was left-over.

Wildlife (and roadkill)

Early in the ride, I also wondered whether the closest I'd come to seeing some American wildlife was an exotic spread of road-kill. I slalomed through squashed raccoons, deer (one enormous one, I assumed to be an elk?), squirrels, possums, chipmunks, snakes and even skunks (which stank as much as I'd read as a boy). I went past what looked to me like large porcupine (do they exist in California?) and an armadillo (again, is that even possible?!). Slowly though these cadavers did make way for more uplifting sights although, initially, these were only drip-fed through: at first, I heard the raucous bark of some distant sea-lions; then, when I saw the black spots of seals out on a rock, they registered as no more than specks to my telescopic camera lens.

Even the early sighting of whales spurting out plumes of water ended up being a rather deflating encounter: with the jolly tone of someone that had spent too long in my own company I had gate-crashed a guided group of whale watchers, when asked if I knew what I was looking for, I quipped, "Something like a big fish....?!" My humour with met with such deadpan distain that I reversed my bike back out onto the road somewhat crestfallen that I'd lost the ability to communicate with my own species.

By the end of the trip, though, I'd had to cover my face as I rode through a flapping wake of vultures picking at food at the roadside; stood pin-drop-quiet within touching distance of a group of deer; and even accidently created a road-kill of my own as I rode straight over a sun-basking snake, despite my best efforts to jump it. I'd watched raccoons and chipmunks steal food from a veranda where I sat, as humming birds buzzed around them and I'd photographed big herds of wild elk (although this did involve pushing aside other tourists to get a line of sight). The scariest wildlife was, perhaps, best left to hints and suggestion: road-signs revealed the presence of bears and coyotes but the closest I got was hearing the tale that a cyclist had ridden into a bear only two weeks earlier and had a broken arm to show for it.

Navigation

In the early stages of the tour, I began to wonder whether I was destined to be stuck on larger highways throughout, but those early thoughts soon became distant concerns. The ride took me on a sliding scale of minor roads, down to the far end of the spectrum where the tarmac disappeared and the surface turned, firstly, to gravel, and then to sand.

Highway 101 was the main artery of the route and, at times, it was a big, brash speedway but I was often grateful to it for sucking away some fast miles.

Highway 1 was its little brother. The not so big, not quite so brash, tributary often dipped closer to the cliffs and waves and ducked through smaller towns less brazenly.

Then there were all those other roads that weren't deemed deserving of a number. These were nearly always the most scenic but were also the most haphazard.

Navigation could have been made easy by just staying on the 101 but that would have meant ten days on a dual carriage-way so I took the detours in good humour.

I only got badly lost once: predictably as I was trying to escape the conurbation of San Francisco. I found myself, firstly, trying to climb a single-track Mountain Bike circuit, as several riders descended at break-neck speed towards me; then, potentially more seriously, at the entrance to a long road tunnel having just passed a sign that stated, "Cyclists take alternate route".

Following a tiny pink line of a cycling GPS computer has its own drawbacks, and bonuses. A couple of times I emerged from the deep cover of inland forests to suddenly find myself atop an ocean cliff and, on one occasion, I did so at such pace that I almost found myself through the barrier before I could compute my surprise that I'd hit the coast.

On my first day, as if to dispel any danger of overconfidence in my whereabouts in the world, I rode past a concentration of tobacco stores – reminiscent of a tax-dodging border crossing – before I passed a "Welcome to Oregon" sign. All very well, although I hadn't realised that I'd ever left that state...

Culture

The towns, like the roads, changed in character the further South I went.

In North Oregon, the flatter coastal plain lent itself to enormously long bridges as the 101 traversed over one river mouth after another.

A couple of these constructions looked like a packet of drinking straws held together with blue-tack. It was as though they'd been built by arguing factions, so dramatically their style changed half way across.

The many inlets held towns trying themselves to bridge a gap between half fishing industry; half tourist-chique. Some cafes were staffed by hipsters straight out of Portland; others, more aligned to the rough and tumble of industrial fishermen.

As the shoreline steepened into more pronounced bays, surfers, and surfing competitions appeared. I sat eating my morning porridge, amongst young athletes squeezed into their own versions of lycra cladding and reflected on how much cooler surfers were compared to an equivalent set of breakfasting audaxers. The scene reminded me of "Point Break" and, later, I had the smug satisfaction of finding out that the film had indeed been shot there. Descending into such bays, the roads often became awash with sand and I tip-toed ever so carefully on my bike.

It wasn't until I approached San Francisco that a new type of culture appeared. Roadside diners started to air their menus in Spanish and the oatmeal and omelettes of my early days were replaced by burritos and fajitas. The price of burritos plummeted from a $13 hipster snack to a $5 working lunch served in a dense wrap the size of my own forearm. Fellow customers ordered in Spanish and smiled politely at our limited exchanges.

Unlike the majority of other cyclo-tourers I met, I was not camping. Instead, I was holing up in the cheapest accommodation I could find each night, usually booked on "Airbnb". The eclectic range of places I lay my head could be a book onto themselves. During the trip I checked in to a: campsite, mobile home, flat, condo, garage, farmhouse, motel, cottage and RV site. Some came with warm hospitality, others did not, but all I needed was a bed and a shower... although perhaps I'd give some a better review than others (!)

Forest and farmland

Although the sea was the predominant feature, my route did have its other chapters: forests, farmlands and even desert (which I'll come on to). And unlike the day rides I'm used to doing around Bristol, these were huge tracts of land that I didn't just shoot past, but I rode through for mile after mile.

The Redwood Pines – and their national park – took me two days. Simplistically a day and a half of steady climbing, then one great, rushing descent. Much of this time was spent in the chasm between vast tree trunks (and through the famous "drive-through-tree"). The feel of the air was almost magical: windless, still and silent; the smell of the pines; and their dappled light. These trees did indeed feel like giants, "The Avenue of the Giants" an apt name. Here the roads were emptier too. On the morning of the long descent I barely saw another vehicle.

As I passed through the forest on the tarmac, I pondered how magical the woods must have been just 100 metres to either side. I felt dwarfed even on my well-trodden road.

Even the intimidating passage of large logging trucks left behind, not the smell of polluting diesel, but the scent of resin and timber – not unlike a five-star sauna.

For me, these were the highlight of my trip. I was moving from A to B at the pace set by my itinerary but this was the area that most demanded to be revisited.

Only 30 miles inland and the feel of the country was very different. Whenever I left the cooling breezes of the coast, the temperatures quickly rose from the comfortable low 20s to above 30. Rather than the ascents being little and often, they became more substantial as I flirted with the mountain ranges parallel to the sea. Nearer to San Francisco, I passed through ranch country and saw groups of actual cowboys, riding actual horses, with actual lassoes. It crossed my mind that they were probably tourists on a "cowboy tour" but I took a photo of the dusty ranch lands in the background and a huge long chain of single file, brown cattle plodding across the dry grasslands.

I was served by a man wearing a T Shirt: "#1 gun safety rule? OWN ONE"; flies attacked me when I stopped, and for the first time I began to run out of water before I reached the next town.

I stayed the night in an "RV Site" on a simple mattress. My host's vest read "My momma told me I could be whatever I wanted? I chose to be an ASSHOLE."

I could now tick-off a couple of Simpsons characters from my list of must-see America.

Tricky to articulate, but it felt as though the locals were used to tougher times and had less indulgence for a cyclo-tourist visiting their town just for fun.

Where the inland was flatter, crop farming displaced the cattle. Enormously vast irrigated fields stretched as far as I could see. Perfectly coiffeured rows of grapes, asparagus, lettuce, artichokes and sod (turf) filled the air with their respective scents. The roads here were incredibly flat, and remarkably straight. But, perhaps surprisingly, my speeds never seemed to rise on these stretches. There was no shelter from the winds and the surfaces were grainy compared to the highways, but in two days of riding I never felt boredom at their repetition. I found myself fascinated at the never-ending rows of geometric precision and the sheer scale of production

Bike and body

As I type out these experiences, I reflect that these intermittent sights are the punctuation points which gave my trip structure. They are the chapter headers, the paragraph breaks and the full-stops. The binding agent, and the flow of the whole trip, was, of course, the riding of my bike. My itinerary comfortably allowed for detours and photo-opportunities; espresso-stops and shopping trips; but also demanded steady progress. I set my alarm at 5.30am every day and was on the road soon after 6. I typically would start to set up for the night around 12-13 hours later; get a shower; clean my bike; then chill out for barely 15 minutes before sleep.

Over and over again I'd do a mental checklist of body and bike:

Bike: tyre feeling a tad soft; brakes perhaps slightly misaligned. A gear or two grating; a strange creaking,perhaps from the seat post? The headset needed retightening; the tri bars had come slightly loose; a bottle-cage was rattling.

Body: my right metatarsal niggled away; my left achilles began to grow sore. My calf muscles took turns in feeling fatigued and needing a stretch; and, by the end of my trip, both my knees were worsening with tendonitis.

I was very consciously focussing my diet on proteins – yoghurts, shakes, bars and chicken burritos - and as the days went past I grew in confidence that I'd get the mileage done.

Eat right, sleep right.

I was eating over 6,000 calories a day and making sure that I slept for eight hours a night.

Perhaps I'd learned these necessities the hard-way on previous tours but, riding on my own, these were easy rules to follow. I could follow every whim of my appetite and body-clock when and as I wanted. After a few days, I'd built up a fairly dependable daily pattern consisting of a large breakfast, mid-morning coffee, early lunch, a mid-afternoon sugar stop, then a large dinner, with further snacks after I'd found a bed for the night. During the course of my tour I actually lost 2.5kg but, overall, I feel that this was a healthy weight-loss, rather than a physical deterioration.

A strained muscle deep in my right thigh caused the greatest concerns. Early in the tour I strapped it once, then twice, and eventually added a third bandage before that pain started to subside around Days 4 and 5. My right hip hurt periodically (probably linked) and my lower back during extended periods in an aero position. Shoulders and neck grew stiff and my biceps tired when the road surface was poor. The palms of my hands developed tender blisters and my wrists went numb. Despite slightly obsessive application of suncream, the back of my neck, cheeks and knees all burned in the sun, and the left side of my face and scalp bristled with an MS-tingle that felt like shingles. I got a toothache and a sore throat. My saddle sores steadily worsened with each passing mile. On one day, I had to pick out a large fly from my right eye and smarted for hours afterwards.

I listened to them all. Adapted where possible. Assessed their messages, and split hairs between complaint and damage.

I don't like drugs, anti-inflammatories or painkillers, believing that they distort messages you need to hear, but, on my final day, I succumbed to the whining from my knees and took some ibuprofens.

This wasn't a race. This was a quest for steady progress. I just had to keep my arms around the various risks at play.

Desert

As I planned my route, the one day that stuck out most ominously was just south of San Francisco. Because a landslide that had closed the coastal road, I was forced inland, through the desert from Salinas to Paso Robles. I was nervous about the distance (my longest day), the climbing (weighteded entirely to the end of the day) and the temperatures (which were likely to be in the mid-30s).

Although that day indeed proved to be the toughest, as so often with cyclo-touring, the greatest challenge was actually an unexpected one and it brought me as close to quitting as I got.

Advised against the 101 for this stretch, I had picked a route on minor roads, but, although I diligently started very early to try to mitigate the day's heat, their cracked and ruptured surfaces almost brought me to my knees. It felt as though I was riding over a sea of cobbles that went on and on, mile after mile, as the sun rose ominously in the sky and the temperatures rose. My speed on the flat dropped to 11... 10... On occasion, I'd hit a stretch of resurfaced road and, with no greater effort, would accelerate up to 18... 19... before hitting the cracks again and dropping right back down.

The juddering road was slowly breaking me.

I stopped at a railroad crossing and to my delight ticked off another couple of my must-sees. Firstly, a steel Amtrak passenger train creaked past. Then a the huge long snake of a commercial goods train. It groaned and squealed past for carriage after carriage, perhaps a mile long.

Then, after I'd barely seen a car all day, a utility truck drove past. On its flatbed was a pile of inflatable rubber rings and two bikini clad women (one wore the stars and stripes – tick). They hollered at me – "Hey baby!!" – before leaving me in their dust (perhaps they were heading to LA as well?) That was enough to bring back the humour to my predicament. I pushed on to Paso Robles and was soon ordering a large iced coffee as I sat by its lush green, irrigated town square.

The finish

If San Francisco hung on my experience of riding over the iconic Golden Gate Bridge (anything from Hitchcock's "Vertigo" to

Michael Bay's "The Rock"), my arrival in LA was the procession of iconic place names and beaches as I rode into movieland.

The ocean road (fact) felt plucked straight from the opening credits of "Big Little Lies" (myth) and the seafront houses grew in glamour and glitz. I thought of Sharon Stone's sea-top mansion from Basic Instinct, and I passed through Malibu, Santa Monica, Venice & Muscle Beaches, and – yes – I saw the Hollywood letter-boards. I can't even remember which, or how many films, I've seen them in before but the beach towers were quintessentially Baywatch and I took a photo of their wide expanses of sand.

I'd spent so many hours in relative seclusion, meditating and day-dreaming, that the busy LA roads felt pretty foreign and jarring.

For days I'd been able to smooth over all the many mental stresses of my life: I'd rolled them over and over in my mind – like pebbles in the Pacific swash – until their rough edges had smoothed, smoothed, then smoothed away. Some disappeared entirely, none jarred anymore.

I'd got to a state of inner peace that I've rarely known before. Left in the isolated bubble of my own devices, my yin and yang were more balanced than ever. Past regrets, future stresses, hopes and fears had all dissipated and I felt a sadness at having to leave this new equilibrium.

The tour was coming to an end: car horns sounded in the LA streets and my reveries were about to be sucked back into the chaos of a shared, real life.

My old friend opened his front door and smiled.

I lent my black bike against the white-washed walls of his garage and took up his offer of a cold can of ginger ale.

This was where the cycling stopped.

The Pacific Coast.

Unforgettable stuff.

The Pacific Coast:
an abstract and an epilogue

Abstract

At the beginning of my journey down the Pacific Coast, I stood in my friend's house in Portland, Oregon, and looked at the huge map of America he had on his wall.

I'd been used to seeing America on the miniature globe on my desk; on this large scale, I'd only ever seen it split into abbreviated day-by-day chunks on my laptop screen.

At this new, wall-sized, explosion, the distances suddenly looked all the more intimidating. Even my very first day's ride, planned to arrive at a dot labelled "Manzanita", looked huge. I could see a long list of towns I'd be passing through. What had seemed like a simple journey along a couple of highways, was now a patchwork of intersections, county and state lines, bays, borders and bridges.

When I (again) checked the internet for last minute tips and weather forecasts, I happened across the site of an adventure company offering organised tours of a similar route.
"93% of our riders agreed that this tour was 'the best thing that they have ever done' "
Ever?
I baulked at the statement (it reminded me of similar claims I had read when trying to find a wedding venue, "100% of our

couples say that their wedding with us was one of the best days of their lives"!)

Suffering from the jet-lag of my transworld flight, I set off in pitch dark the following morning. Almost immediately I missed a turn and found myself riding on a giant overpass as commuting traffic squeezed past me at speed.

Carefully does it... a long way still to go.

The best thing ever? Let's see.

Ten and a half days later I slowly rolled up to the front door of my friend's house in LA.

I uncleated my shoes, stopped my ride computer and took a few deep breaths.

My arms and legs were buzzing slightly with tiredness.

My face was glowing with wind and sunburn and I'd grown a wilderness beard.

I'd cycled 1,650 miles.

Along the coast. Through Redwood Forests. Across a desert. Over a mountain range.

My journey was now at an end.

Epilogue

Now I'm back in Bristol, back at my desk and back at work.

At this exact point in time, another cyclist will probably be setting out from the Canadian border, making his or her way south.

Another "me" will be stopping to take another photo of the Golden Gate Bridge, probably from the exact same viewpoint.

Somewhere they'll be some other rider, leaning on their bike, trying to summon up those last energy reserves to ride that last 10, 20... 50 miles for the day;

But for two weeks, that had been me. *Living the dream*.

Of course, my rolling up to a friend's house in LA wasn't "The End". Nothing stopped at that arbitrary line in the sand. Neither was my pitch-dark departure "The Beginning". Before that there had been the flight from Heathrow... the drive to the airport... and the booking of the trip some eight months ago.

There was that trip to the USA in 2005, that I'd planned but never took place.

There was the map of the world on my bedroom wall when I was still at school, complete with pins where I'd been and where I'd wanted to go.

And a generation ago, there was my Granny, riding her fixed gear bike in the Cairngorms of Scotland, up the hill to Tomintoul. Before my dad... before he met my mum... before me.

And there was me in Southmead Hospital in March 2015, digesting the fact that I'd just been diagnosed with MS.

Me, holding back my emotions as I tried to cycle down the hill to work with barely enough the strength to lift my legs... and me, trying to cycle up the Col du Tormalet as my perceptions of dreams and reality blurred.

Me, lying on the kitchen floor as my body swirled with vertigo, recovering from my second bout of chemotherapy.

And me and my nadir: being lifted to my feet by a cinema usher as my distorted senses left me unable to leave my chair.

Time existed before, and time will continue to do so.

But those two weeks did feel like a moment apart.

A wash of memories and landscapes; emotional highs and lows that I will ring-fence as something special.

And – yeah – I'd tick that box: it might actually have been the best thing I've ever done.

So, back in Bristol, back at my desk and back at work.

A friend has recommended a book called "After the ecstasy, the laundry".

The next day of now.

I look at some of the photos I took. Somehow none of them quite seem to capture the real essence of the trip – another beach; another view – snapshots in time that don't quite describe the whole journey.

1,650 miles of cycling but perhaps the real challenge is when the riding ends.

Chapter Ten: What does it all mean?

Where is cycling taking me?

I've long ridden bikes. I've explored, commuted, travelled and toured, but it was only a few years ago that I entered my first "time trial" event. I turned up on my old steel bike, wearing mountain biking shoes, gym shorts and a cagoule. I couldn't really believe what I'd stumbled upon. In an otherwise completely non-descript A-road lay-by, there was a collection of lyra-clad riders warming-up on static rollers. They had bikes that looked like shining carbon spaceships, they wore weird pointy helmets and had gnarly body shapes that looked like snakes. I might have been imagining it but even their faces seemed streamlined and honed. The organiser encouraged me to remove my billowing waterproof before I started but I didn't like the thought of riding through drizzle so parachuted my way around as young whippets shot past, tucked into their aero positions.

Several people were friendly, although it was fairly clear that I wasn't "one of them". I definitely wasn't one of the cool kids. Some seemed to distance themselves from my dishevelment as if it might be contagious to their sleekness. I imagine that the organiser would probably not have bet on seeing me again, but I turned up again the following week, having fitted road tyres to my bike and dispensed with my jacket. The same friendly faces made small talk with me and encouraged me to keep going.

Some of those guys will have been breaking themselves training through winter: indoor spin classes, leg weights and chain-gangs of head-down cyclists in the rain. I perhaps understand a bit more now about how they saw me when I first turned up: I was fresh from commuting to work on my bike and only when the sun shone. Keen but green, I was friendly but somehow had a lot to learn. And my bike could have done with a clean.

A few weeks later, I tried to join an unofficial club ride during the week. The route was very hilly and I got dropped almost immediately. About an hour later, the group screamed past me as they descended in the completely opposite direction: I was lost, they were lapping me and I was probably in their way.

Early on my recent 600km audax, I found myself riding alongside a guy I'd met several times before (the pool of cyclists that enter these crazy events is probably pretty small). I retain his anonymity – let's call him "Steve" – but he is quite a personality on the audax circuit. He rides further, faster and more frequently than virtually anyone else. I wondered if he still enjoyed all those miles. This event was definitely a spectacular one – over Snowdonia and through the Beacons – but many are not so, designed instead to make the miles obtainable. Typically, long audax routes focus on being flat and steady rather than spectacular. Mile after mile, or, in his case, mile after mile after mile. A pleasure? Hobby? Love? Or an obsession? I know, for sure, that he earns those miles. Often riding solo, he rarely drafts behind other riders. More often than not, it's him pulling others forward.

One of the frustrations of such long-distance events is the etiquette of riding with others. Some sit silently on your back wheel for mile after mile as you act as their unacknowledged windbreak. There are no rules being broken, other than those of fairness and honour. "Steve" was growling to me, perhaps more to himself, as a group tucked in behind us. It was as though he had earned his place at these events the hard way – the proper way – and he resented all those others getting away with an easy ride. Our speeds, then paths, deviated as he knuckled down into another event. Another one he'd ticked off, tutting at the pretenders who couldn't do it on their own accord.

Amongst groups trying to cope tough, there will always be some who are already tougher than others. In his eyes, I doubt some of us even qualify as cyclists.

I got a place in the Welsh Velothon through a friend. It's a 90-mile route from Cardiff with the massive attraction of being on closed (i.e. car-free) roads. It's a huge event. Around 10,000 cyclists wend their way around at their different speeds, with their different outlooks, attitudes, approaches and ambitions.

I was looking forward to the closed roads – nothing beats sweeping round blind corners knowing that nothing is going to be coming the other way – but my allocated start time was right at the very back of the field. I'd done events like this before *(see "La Maratona"),* sabotaged by thousands of cyclists in front of me who prevent any momentum, rhythm, or speed.

The buzz at the start was infectious, but, as I rolled off, the congestion of cyclists on the road was marked. The early miles on the flat were completely navigable but as the first inclines appeared and the roads narrowed, progress got more haphazard. Some riders were stopping to walk, others were zigzagging with effort. I was overtaking most but every so often someone would shoot past me on my right, "COMING THROUGH". A torrential cloud-burst then soaked the field. I rode past several prostrate crash victims – one in a brace; another under an emergency space blanket. Visibility deteriorated as I spent more and more time hugging the right-hand verge, wanting to keep my tempo, but not wanting to crash trying.

I came into contact with another cyclist as we briefly rode abreast; he slipped over and his swerve took me down as well. Nothing serious but the roads felt chaotic, full of first-time cyclists and slippery on my misjudged slick tyres.

Guys in overpriced kit, pushed incredibly expensive bikes up the steeper hills. There's never much dignity in pushing a bike, especially in cleats. I couldn't help but wonder what they were doing – all the gear; but no steel. No miles and miles on the road, their bikes bought, then kept in bubble wrap in the garage.

I type this in what feels like the year's first week of sun.

I've taken to joining a group of cyclists in Central Bristol that meet up for a quick lunchtime ride during the week, "Lunch Club".

Sometimes I'm the only person that turns up but this week, with a larger group, was particularly pleasurable. Short sleeves and shorts; warm weather and us riding in time.

Conversation was in snippets, we took turns in the front and the ride was quick. The final descent was particularly breathless.

Smiles all round, then back to our respective desks and work. Those guys had become my new friends.

It had just passed 1am.

It was 19 hours since the start and I'd been pedalling for 17 of them.

I hadn't seen anyone else for over an hour. I think there was one, maybe two, riders ahead of me.

It was near freezing and my hands and feet were numb. The stars were quite stunning. The cold, crisp air was certainly clear.

I had stopped to try and connect my charger to my GPS unit which was almost out of power, but my hands were struggling with the fiddling wires.

I was pleased that I had my woollen snood with me. Pleased that I'd packed my warmer gloves.

I was going to stop and sleep in less than 10 kilometres time.

I felt invigorated, excited and incredibly alive. Very tired, but happy.

MS was nowhere near me.

I don't know where cycling is going to take me. I can't even work out where it's taken me from, but it does give me *something*. Maybe not all a good *thing*, but certainly a *thing* that is not MS.

With hindsight you can see yourself through other's eyes. It is harder to do the same in the present.

I hope I can instil in my boys the thoughts that however fast you think you are, there is always someone faster; no matter how slow you think you are, there is always someone slower. It's good to see both sides of that coin: never be too proud, nor too self-conscious.

What type of cyclist do I want to be?

Professional cyclists have long enjoyed heavily-tailored, scientific performance plans. Training zones, VO2 levels, hematocrit scores and measures of residual exhaustion. Peaking and recovering – anaerobic, aerobic – and lactate thresholds.

These seems a world away from the trundling commuters I follow down the Bristol-Bath cycle-path to work. Rather than aero-fit, lightweight mesh-suits, they wear bobble hats, ski gloves and work-boots. They ride ill-fitted mountain bikes with slow flat tyres, carry packed lunch rucksacks, rattling, heavy D-locks and fading & muddied rear lights.

Lunch Club on a Wednesday continues to be a bit hit and miss. Sometimes I'm the only attendee, other days there have been ten of us chafing at the bit in the sun. One of my friends has turned up a few times on his off-the-shelf road bike (read sporty-looking, but built to be robust, rather than fast). He's happy to carry the unimposing air of a desk-working commuter, donning a flapping windproof, out for a social chat in his lunch hour. I enjoy his company and, although a strong cyclist, he is relaxed if he gets slightly left behind on some of the steeper hills.

This summer he also set a new club record for a team 30 mile time trial.

Photos of this ride reveal a scarcely recognisable bike... and man. His gleaming carbon race bike, the black frame unbroken by either decal or logo, fairly drips with speed; his wheels' spokes have been replaced by expensive looking solid discs; and the forward pointing, horizontal handlebars look about a foot too low to be comfortable. Even his water-bottle is a strange, streamlined shape, tucked neatly away to avoid ruining his lines.

His all-in-one skin-suit looks like a tattoo (*eyes up, ladies*), and his shoes look as though have been wrapped in bright cling-film to better slip through the air. His helmet looks as if molten plastic has been dripped onto his head as he entered a wind tunnel. Even his gloves look as though they've been painted on.

He knows what all racing cyclists know. That lunch clubs are not there to race. Overtakes on the Bristol Cyclepath en route to work shouldn't be a cause of satisfaction.

If you want to race, train to race.... then race.

But to race at this level (/his level) doesn't come cheap. Nor, of course, do these levels of fitness and power come easy.

Consider, though, how any quest for self-improvement blurs the two:

The fairest, truest times are against yourself – same bike, same conditions - from a week before. Or a month ago. Or from last year. The challenge here is one of "self-improvement", to see how you can get your body to best evolve to the demands you make of it.

For my part, I've spent many weeks entering time-trials ("TTs") ridden around Chew Valley Lake, trying to chisel down a faster time, whilst acknowledging the variances in wind speeds and direction, isobars, humidity and so on *(et cetera et cetera ad infinitum)*.

I was enjoying the challenge and was shaving down my time by handfuls of seconds but then I bought some cheap, clip-on "tri-bars" which hold you, the cyclist, in a more unbroken aero-position, and my PB dropped by over a minute (out of a total of 22) overnight.

I should have felt delighted... but, strangely, this was the point that my interest in time-trialling began to dwindle. Progress began to feel like a factor of how much money I was willing to spend.

Last week I watched a documentary called "Man Vs Snake": one man's journey to set a computer high-score. This was not just to be his own PB, or the best ever score on his computer, but the best score ever in the whole world, out of everyone that had ever played the game. I suppose, this is the crux of these quests for self-improvement; at some point, you wonder how your "self-improvement" compares to everyone else's. For these are the arenas where glories are won – in bird's nest stadiums, public leaderboards and trophy rooms - not within mental notes-to-self regarding week-to-week differences on sociable, club TTs. And the problem with these public arenas is that others can spend their money on all the lighter-weight tri-bars; solid disc wheels; and molten-plastic-dripped helmets that they can buy.

In the world of professional cycling, a willingness to spend money becomes a willingness to add all those other marginal gains. I echo the above: to race at this level doesn't come cheap nor, of course, do these levels of fitness and power come easy. Pros have to tick-off the latter, so that they can be as efficient as possible with the former. Neither this book nor, it seems, the whole internet are big enough to nail down the moral rights and wrongs of Bradley Wiggins' TUE steroidal asthmatic injections but if the "kit" isn't the same, and the "base lines" aren't aligned, how can efforts at self-improvement be fairly compared? How can I be expected to keep up with that guy riding a carbon space-ship?

Last winter, amongst my cycling friends in Bristol, a new device was in town.

When roads freeze over and rains come down, there is always a retreat to indoor spin classes and garage-based turbo trainers but this year the craze seemed to explode. Because indoor bikes can now be linked up to laptops and the internet, cyclists can "race" friends, avatars and other assorted pixelated AI-creations around any famous course or climbs that they can imagine, all without going outside.

My friends bought indoor trainers and my friends got fast.

They could assess their threshold levels, heart rate zones and suffer scores, data that were once the preserve of the pros.

And it worked.

At the same time, I'd be slowly riding my commuting bike with its knobbly tyres, in the rain, fretting about my pins and needles.

But, when the winter skies were clear, it was me that got to see Orion's Belt in the early morning darkness.

Some of the scenes from the Rocky films still stick with me from my child-hood. In Rocky II (paraphrasing from imdb.com): *Rocky's boxing-foe, Drago, scientifically uses high-tech lab equipment, steroid enhancement and has a team of trainers and doctors monitoring his every movement. Rocky, on the other hand, throws heavy logs, chops down trees, pulls an overloaded snow sleigh, jogs in heavy snow and treacherous icy conditions and climbs a mountain.*

The film leaves the viewer in no doubt as to the romance of the two approaches.

But maybe, amongst all the other suspensions of disbelief you're asked to hold for their final fight, the fact that Rocky actually triumphs despite the above is perhaps the least believable. The film's message is that it is Rocky who has the soul, not the science.

Back to CyclingWithMS.

It has become cycling when I can.

When I can, I cycle fast.

When I can't, I am relieved I can still ride my bike.

I race myself on hills where I know my PBs.

I fight my MS when it tells me I'm weak.

And when I race new found friends at Lunch Club as they don their heavy commuting shoes, billowing wind-sheets and cyclo-cross bikes, I don't forget who my real race is against.

Winning is being there, on my bike, for another day.

When I'm forced off my bike, I need to learn to remember that there are bigger things at play. This is when I struggle to escape the feeling that I'm getting spat out the back. Life is so much easier when you're cruising at the same speed as the peloton surround.

Samurai Cycling

Cycling is, for the vast majority, a hobby and a way to breathe in fresh air.

Of course, it's also a way from A to B and, if I'm philosophising, not necessarily just geographically (see the last chapter).

But, although it can offer reflections on life, it rarely becomes a way of life in itself: it is a pastime, not a religion (although I have seen amusing cycling T-shirts proclaiming "I worship at the altar of the handlebars" and "My only religion is cycling").

That said, to fully embrace something – to dedicate energy to any pursuit or goal or to work towards an aspiration or ambition – must encourage some reflections as to the meaning of life: how it can be best enjoyed and whether or not your current choices are allowing that. Thoughts expand beyond the activity itself – be it marathon training or revising for an exam – to encompass what you eat and drink, how you plan and organise your time & commitments and how & when you interact with others - indeed what others may think about your latest choices.

You may be familiar with David Brailsford. As Performance Director of the Sky Cycling Team, he made his name, and the name of British Cycling, through an attention to detail that surpassed all others. Main keystone events are revered and worked around. His athletes are prepared physically, psychologically and emotionally through tweaks to their training, diets and minds, all leading up to a single moment in time when it should all come to fruition. Behind the scenes, focus will not necessarily have been about the velodrome tself, but will have encompassed everything from the type of polish on the floor to the grain of the floorboards:

Every detail has a purpose, demanding contemplation, appreciation and, then, understanding. It is through their study, that such details take on different forms, until even the grains of the floorboards can be described as having a personality and beauty of their own.

In this way, it is interesting, and paradoxical, that the greater the singularity of focus, the greater the need for a wider appreciate of everything else...

...which brings me round to the **Samurai.**

From the moment they woke, they devoted themselves to the perfection of whatever it was that they pursued. Although the Bushido (their code of conduct) stated that loyalty, courage, veracity, compassion, and honour were important above all else, an appreciation and respect of life were also considered imperative, as this added the necessary balance to a warrior's character. Be it the making of tea, the application of make-up or their sword-craft, the samurai were encouraged to appreciate, understand and absorb the strength and beauty that existed all around them and to be disciplined in their approaches to nature and to life.

In Julian Barnes "History of the World in 10 1/2 Chapters", there is a tale about heaven. A golfer there enjoys steady and continuous improvement at his game, until the point is reached when he can card a round of 18 shots. The problem (I paraphrase) is that he started to miss the strains of achievement from the real world. There was no celestial golfing equivalent of winter miles in the hail, a punctured rear tyre in a heavy downpour or the risk of (another) calorie-misjudgement vaporising your leg-power with 30 miles still to go. The ambitions that are most satisfying are the ones that are hardest earned.

When we lived in Australia a few years ago I dabbled at golf myself. To my embarrassment, upon entering a local match-play tournament, I came head-to-head with one of the most experienced luminaries of the WA Golfing scene.

With only two holes left of our game, solely because of my (very appropriately high) handicap, I was faced with a short four-foot putt directly up a steep hill which would win the hole… but I also knew that two-putts would draw. Rather embarrassingly, but completely typically, despite having one of the safest shots the game can offer, I left my first putt well short, but was still satisfied when I sunk my second attempt. But my opponent was genuinely upset at this performance. It took a me a while to understand such an apparently disproportionate reaction: he had happily tolerated my complete failure to adhere to the most inclusive of dress-codes *(with hindsight, not something I'm proud of)*; he had appreciated, rather than depreciated, my use of cheap, second-hand clubs; and had not been offended by the wear and tear shown by my aged golf-balls. But my putting strategy, I now realise, was seen as a betrayal of the game he loved, a lack of attention to detail and to one of the most basic fundamentals of the sport. Worse still, it implied that I could turn up to play against him with disregard and a lack of focus. He took it as a sign of disrespect to his own efforts, preparation and training that I could be so castaway with my own attempts.

He won the last hole, knocked me out of the tournament and went on to qualify for the state-wide final.

It has been a while since I have actively trained at cycling - "practise with the objective of enhancing performance". MS has too frequently nullified events that I have been focussing on, so, instead, I cycle when I can, go fast when my health allows and am satisfied to enjoy the scenery when it does not. One blessing of my diagnosis has been my re-evaluation (or re-reflection) of life which had enhanced these experiences: MS has simplified my cycling ambitions and offered a greater clarity (purity?) and perspective of purpose. Sometimes I'm fast, sometimes I'm slow, but I won't beat myself up about it. However, to those that take the sport more seriously – be it through aero-clothing, indoor-training, or more blood, sweat and tears - chapeau to you and my respect to your efforts.

And as for Samurai Cycling? I do like my friend's recent ride-title on Strava: "Lunch Ride with a pause for martial arts training session in the woods", but, as perhaps a better example: I recently emailed a cyclist from my club who had just found a new off-road route up one of Bristol's more iconic climbs. He is a national-level rider so I was half-expecting a response filled with cassette-gearing and HR zones (he had set the fastest time ever ridden up that hill) but he replied: "Watch out for the sequoia trees on the right, they're just coming into yellow flower."

Samurai Cycling indeed.

Reflections

They say time flies when you're having fun...so last week I had my first consultant MS check-up, post-lemtrada.

Actually, it was with the registrar and was nigh on six months late, but my MS-birthday was dutifully celebrated.

MS is no longer a shock nor an excitement. I'm still naive as to what MS means for my future – of course, no one know what's around the corner – but I am now one year closer to knowing what'll happen for the rest of my life.

Hopefully, if I live to 90, I'm barely only 2% of the way to a true understanding of my MS. I like the thought of me dropping off to sleep in the year 2066 with the sudden thought, "So, that's what it meant when I was diagnosed..."

Things are becoming clearer, at least, more familiar. I'm not sure that this makes me any wiser but my initial thoughts and advice received are both now largely bearing themselves out. It feels like I'm now experiencing what was previously just an academic exercise.

Upon diagnosis I wrote:

"The causes, symptoms and prognoses for MS sufferers (I now know) are difficult to sum up succinctly. You've basically got an issue – unique to yourself – which you're going to have to live with for the rest of your (hopefully long) life and manage as best you can.

It's not curable.

It could be very bad. Could be not-so-bad...

Its development can be managed with diet and drugs. As to the exact path it takes? You are, to some extent, in the lap of the Gods (but, then again, aren't we all?) It would be extremely dangerous to ignore it, but it is something you can live around, or force to live around you, albeit with fingers crossed."

Several years later, I don't think I can really add too much to that but, if I could go back in time and talk to the pre-diagnosis "me", there are maybe a few thoughts I'd like to share:

- Firstly, be enormously grateful for the diagnosis itself. Not only because of the pharmaceutical, chemotherapy and treatment options that it entails but because of its impacts socially and maritally. I hope I'm not going around begging pity or sympathy, but such a diagnosis offers a crutch to explain those unannounced bouts of vertigo, those disproportionate waves of tiredness and fatigue, my abstention from alcohol and careful early nights. Weird bouts of listlessness or post-viral exhaustion are no longer met with such frustration because I now have a genuine excuse (*"O pity the patient"*). The first people I told of my diagnosis, I felt like I was letting in to some big secret but, now, I can talk about it matter-of-factly, aware that it really is not that big a deal *(touch wood)* and barely registers as a dot on most people's days
- Secondly, living with MS is increasingly bearing itself out as a psychological battle, rather than physical one. I have never been in bad pain *(touch wood again),* my MS is more of a millstone of niggles, discomforts and feeling crap. These are symptoms that I can live with – socialise with, work with, cycle with and even laugh with – but they demand to be hit head-on by a never-ending positivity. I have to keep smiling, despite the crap. It's when the doubts creep in and I struggle to lift myself, that the millstone has weighed heavy. When my spirit has needed some sleep and the adrenalin has run

dry, MS has proved tough. At times, I've reached points when I've just had enough of too many, and such incessant, low level niggles and discomforts. Residual symptoms, by definition, are there the whole time so, strictly, they impact everything. Glass half-full, they ruin nothing; glass half-empty, they ruin everything.

- And, thirdly, believe what you feared, MS is indeed an unlucky thing to have but it's not *that* bad. Things could be so much worse. The things that others have to live with make me embarrassed should I make any fuss, or should any fuss be made of me. When I was diagnosed I kept asking, "but what's so bad about it?" "If it's not so bad, when I tell people about it why do they react with shock?" The truth is somewhere in between because it is bad and shocking, surprising news to absorb, but this is largely because I still appear to be so healthy and far removed from disability. It would be more worrying if the news were expected.
- MS has sharpened the joy that I feel and my enthusiasm for seeking it out. It's given me more perspective as to what matters and removed any feelings of self-conscience about who I am and how my body works. I can now face up to one of my issues that had been hiding for so long and dispense with all those undercurrents of uncertainty and self-doubt: it feels as though my Yin and Yang are now more aligned and I understand myself more.

At times, I still feel as though I have a lot to deal with. Must be the obsessive control freak in me that mulls all these new emotions over and over again until they start to make more sense and feel familiar. I escape out on my bike and the swirling thoughts start to calm into a more orderly flow of currents. Sometimes, though, I cycle and my legs give out before the mental knots have been untied but, even then, the skies remain so huge that my issues still shrink, dwarfed by the outdoors.

There's more to find out and, given time, I'm sure that my new sense of self will have been built anew. But at the moment, I still puzzle about what or who I am: cycling 200 miles with dust and sweat marking the creases in my brow; or suffering the indignity of being sat down by an MS nurse to be shown how to use a catheter. No one said it'd be easy but I ride my bike, value my friends and, despite everything else, I can't really imagine anywhere else I'd rather be.

Perhaps, for now, my work here is done

December 2017

I run the risk of starting off with some pseudophilosophy, but I think we can agree that life has a distinct beginning and, of course, one "Big End". And whatever happens in between, you can't really quarrel with those two points.

I've always written something of a journal. Today, dusty travel-diaries have been replaced by notebook keyboards, websites and blogs. Much of it I don't share, and perhaps I don't always get the balance right: when I re-read past blogs I sometimes find myself embarrassed at their self-obsession and melodrama.

Upon diagnosis, I set about writing this book, unsure of where it would go; but it was meant to provide a sounding board for my own experiences of MS and to offer insights to the similarly recently diagnosed. If they happened to be cyclists, I hoped that they'd find a narrative which, whilst although inevitably different to the stories they would face, would offer them information (and inspiration?) where I had struggled to find the same.

I have now written about the period of my initial diagnosis; two chemotherapy treatments and their aftermath and many of the highs and lows in between.

Now, in December 2017, this is certainly not the Big End, but it feels as though a story – my story – has now run something of a full arc.

Although, again this year, I suffered my annual autumnal malaise, I began to feel that I had reached a stability with my MS and, though this may not be exactly the life I would have chosen

– good health in the summer, with periods of poor health on either side – it is still a life very much worth living. In fact, this last summer, must have been one of the best of my life.

My MS is at times saddening. Disappointing. Frustrating. And on rare occasions, upsetting. Worrying. And, on the odd occasion, defeating.

But this year I have continued to ride my bike and, at times, have felt as healthy as I've ever been.

I await the future, like all of us, but must claim to be happy in the present.

Where I've had to give ground to MS, I like to think that it has always been a considered retreat – inch by inch – rather than a panicked capitulation.

Trying to make the most of the hand still in play.

Whilst, at one level, all bike rides must start, and then finish, it is the want of us cyclists to impose our own arbitrary lines in the sand, to set landmarks to reach or fail / win or lose.

Earlier this year, I wrote about my bike ride down the Pacific Coast of America, but one slight regret I omitted: initially I had planned to ride all the way down to the Mexican border. It had been wholly within reach until a perfect storm of mechanical (cracked seat post) and electronic (broken GPS device and phone) malfunctions had slowed me down as I approached San Francisco. I was never to make up that lost time.

Of course, the ride I did was "my ride", rich with variety, adventure and (self-awarded) glory. But I never quite made it all the way down.

My line in the sand, had crept northwards until LA became my finish line.

I felt the glow of completion; but, also the nagging regret of those last 150 miles left unridden, to some arbitrary line in the sand that I had deemed it necessary to reach.

A refusal to capitulate but coupled with an acknowledgement of changing circumstance and possibility.

Trying to make the most of the hand still in play.

My last touring ride of the year was following the River Rhone, down from Lake Geneva, all the way to the Mediterranean. Southern France was rusting with autumnal colours and, even down through Provence, winter's weather was knocking at the door.

I had planned the route on a somewhat ad hoc basis but was revelling in an anticipated sense of completion, riding a river from source to sea. It was only late on the second day, that my friend pointed out to me that the source of the river was actually several days ride to the North of Lake Geneva. Like the final leg down to Mexico, this was going to have to be conquered another time. Or perhaps another lifetime.

As the river widened towards the coast, at least the saltwater goal of the Med, remained in sight. Until we awoke on the final morning to a howling storm and 50mph winds.

We made it as far down as Arles.

My friend was blown clean off his bike.

Twice a cross wind pushed me off the road and into the verge.

I was hit by a runaway rubbish bin as it was blown towards me like a bowling ball.

One bridge proved impossible to cross. In the end I walked my bike from one side to the next, pausing behind any windbreak I could find.

So the red-line of my ride didn't quite reach the sea.

And riding through heavy rain on the second day meant that I had a serious head cold setting in as we caught the train home.

The next day, my old MS symptoms were blazing and I spent the next few days in bed swaying with a buzzing vertigo and a pulsing muscle ache.

On that occasion, the line in the sand hadn't been pulled back quite fast enough. As I lay in bed, I reflected that it's always better to have a hand in play. Even it's not the one you would necessarily wish for.

The most arbitrary of all my cycling goals is the number of miles I cycle in each calendar year. Luckily, web-based tracking tools do all the work for me, leaving me to ride to the next pointless milestone, which no one else but me will notice.

A few years ago, I wondered if I would ever reach 10,000 km. That became 10,000 miles. Then 12,000. Then 1,000 every month. This year, with no long hospital stays, no chemotherapy treatments and a summer of touring, my running total is 14,300, with 15,000 was very much in my sights.

But I'm now off my bike again, feeling down with MS symptoms nagging away.

So close to a line in the sand that I can almost touch, my eyes flitting between the rich pot and the hand I've been dealt.

No one but me will notice.

But disappointing. Frustrating. And, on rare occasions, upsetting. Worrying.

I must remember to keep adjusting the lines that don't matter so I can still go on and reach the ones that do.

For now, it's LA (not Mexico). Arles (not the Med). 14 (not 15).

When I was diagnosed, I'd already been suffered the cumulating symptoms of MS for five or six years.

Whilst, when I finish this paragraph, I'll be off into the unknown, diagnosis was never the beginning, nor is this the end.

When it asks for a mile, I may give it an inch but I will fight it on the hills in Bristol; and on my tours to Europe and beyond. On club-rides, lunchtime socials, head-down time trials and commutes to work.

I'm lucky to be CyclingWithMS and long may that continue. MS may be a fact, but the cycling bit is still a choice.

Bookend

It's now been two years since my second dose of lemtrada.

The treatment was never sold to me as a cure for my MS. Clinical trials had shown that the drug might reduce the frequency of relapses by 50%, but it wouldn't be to zero.

I try to bear this in mind as I review the last 12 months. I was ill for almost four months between November and March. Never badly so, but I my body seemed to be stuck in an inescapable rut of malaise, vertigo and fatigue.

But then followed a fantastic summer, when I felt as healthy as I'd even been. By September, I had cycled over 10,000 miles, many of them rough, off-road riding on my new adventure-bike.

Later that month though, I had a worrying relapse. If last winter's malaises could maybe attributed to the bad luck of a winter's colds and flu, this was unequivocally a new MS event. For over three weeks, I had almost no feeling from the belly-button down, pin and needles in both arms and hands and a shingle-like tingling that stretched from the top of my head, across my shoulders and down the left hand side of my back.

This annual pattern so closely echoes previous years that, at face-value, it feels as though nothing has really changed, let alone improved, since my lemtrada treatment. What's more, my monthly blood tests still show my lymphocytes struggling to return to their pre-treatment level. But, if there have been some tough months this year, there is a silver-lining: I've been able to turn my ongoing blog posts into this single, coherent book.

Off the bike, off-work and pretty much off-life, I've had the opportunity to finish off a project that I've long aspired to: getting my book written and into published ink. I edited, twisted, contorted and culled many of the blogs that I'd written over the last few years and I'm now content with what is left.

I am happy that this book now tells my story of being diagnosed with MS and of me trying to find a way forward despite it.

Whilst I've been feeling down these last few weeks, re-reading some of my blogs about what I've done these last few years, where I've been and what I've overcome, has helped to remind me of what is possible and that I must stay strong.
I hope that others will feel similarly inspired.

Then, last week, I crashed my bike again. The impact was sufficient to rip one of my shoes into two, crack my helmet and write-off my bike. In fact, only my socks managed to avoid being destroyed. So I type these last sentences staring out the window at blue, sunny skies, nursing a broken wrist, tender with a fuzzy mixture of body-length cuts and bruises.

The outside air, though, does look so very fresh and clear. And is probably perfect weather for cycling.

I still want to get back on my bike and, whilst that remains the case, my belief is that everything else will be OK.

If you would like to contact me or have any feedback or questions about my book, please do feel free to post a message on my blog:

https://cyclingwithms.wordpress.com/

Many thanks to Andrew Prescott for his help with the cover design:

www.andrewprescott.co.uk

Printed in Poland
by Amazon Fulfillment
Poland Sp. z o.o., Wrocław